Thorne's Better Medical Writing

Thorne's
Better Medical Writing

STEPHEN LOCK, MA, MB, FRCP,
Editor, *British Medical Journal*

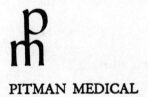

PITMAN MEDICAL

FOR SHIRLEY

First published 1970
Second edition 1977
Reprinted 1977

PITMAN MEDICAL PUBLISHING CO LTD
42 Camden Road, Tunbridge Wells,
Kent TN1 2QD

Associated Companies

UNITED KINGDOM
Pitman Publishing Ltd, London
Focal Press Ltd, London

USA
Fearon-Pitman Publishers Inc, California

AUSTRALIA
Pitman Publishing Pty Ltd, Melbourne

CANADA
Pitman Publishing, Toronto
Copp Clark Publishing, Toronto

EAST AFRICA
Sir Isaac Pitman and Sons Ltd, Nairobi

SOUTH AFRICA
Pitman Publishing Co SA (Pty) Ltd, Johannesburg

NEW ZEALAND
Pitman Publishing NZ Ltd, Wellington

ISBN: 0 272 79413 9
Cat. No. 21 2212 81

Set in 11 pt. Linotype Granjon by
Western Printing Services Ltd, Avonmouth, Bristol.
Printed by offset-lithography and bound
in Great Britain at The Pitman Press, Bath

Contents

Preface to Second Edition

You may say that morality will not benefit from this book. I'm sorry, but people have been fed on sweets too long and it has ruined their digestion. Bitter medicines and harsh truths are needed now, though please don't imagine that the present author was ever vain enough to dream of correcting human vices. Heaven preserve him from being so naïve! It simply amused him to draw a picture of contemporary man as he understands him and as he has, to his own and your misfortune too often found him. Let it suffice that the malady has been diagnosed—heaven alone knows how to cure it!

Lermontov, *A Hero of Our Time*, trans. Paul Foote (Penguin)

As the authors of the first edition of *Better Medical Writing* we (Tony Smith and Stephen Lock) cloaked our identity under the name of one of our favourite characters from Anthony Trollope: as two assistant editors of the *British Medical Journal* we did not want to seem to be committing the *Journal* to a particular line about why articles were accepted or rejected. This is still so: the book is about medical writing in general and not about papers for the *B.M.J.* in particular. But several more recent books on the subject (notably the excellent ones by Calnan and Barrabas and by Woodford and O'Connor) have come to the same general recommendations for writing better articles, and with the present trend away from anonymity we thought that it was time to disclose our identities. In fact, for 'we' the reader should now substitute 'I', for alas, Tony Smith is too pressed with other commitments to help with the new version. Though I am now entirely responsible for the book, I should like to thank him wholeheartedly for his enthusiasm over the first edition—which made it great fun to write—and for his help and criticism of the second.

The natural tendency to expand any first edition should always be resisted: the cautionary tale of a good, single-author, readable, short—and cheap—textbook evolving into an indifferent, multi-author, unreadable, long—and expensive—one is no fable, but a reality, as can be seen by reading any book review columns in a medical journal. Even so, the extra pages in this second edition have been used to repair some of the deficiencies in the first, whether shown by *l'esprit de l'escalier* (infuriatingly obvious as soon as the book was in print), pointed out by reviewers, or disclosed through running courses on medical writing. The most obvious omission, how to write reasonable English, has been corrected by a new chapter on the subject. A second criticism, that Thorne was too limited about British journals and too parochial about overseas ones, has been met by expanding the discussion on the first, but, more importantly, by persuading Dr George Dunea (a British expatriate in Chicago who writes a racy column in the *B.M.J.* every month) to guide us through the choices available among American journals. I have now helped to run 15 courses on medical writing at home and abroad, at most of which Dr Bill Whimster has been a collaborator. Two lessons of these courses are that, however excellently overseas doctors speak English, many of them find it difficult to write; and that, though certain difficulties are peculiar to their nationality, many of these are problems common to all nationalities. So I am sure that many readers will find Dr Whimster's chapter on mistakes commonly made by non-English-speaking writers helpful. But, as every editor knows, medical writing still has a long way to go: unkempt, ill-written articles of ridiculous length still crash through his letter-box every week. The standards of speaking at medical meetings are often better than those of written articles, for at least some organisations such as the Medical Research Society and the Surgical Research Society have strict rules: no paper to be read or to last over 10 minutes, for example.

Some of the rules of medical writing can be taught in two or three lectures to postgraduates, or in a short day's course which also includes, say, advice on speaking at meetings. Even better, or perhaps combined with a course, would be a return to the old system whereby the head of a department personally went through a paper with its junior author. Alas, few of them now have the time for this, and, regrettably, some of them no longer write good articles themselves. Perhaps the ideal solution is for each junior to attend small-group seminars in which papers by him and the other participants are discussed in detail and improved. Editors could help in running these, and also in making things easier for authors, by finally agreeing on a common format for lay-out, figures, tables, and references. For years they have been talking about the need for this; nothing has happened, and yet it is ludicrous that authors should be forced to have their articles that have been rejected by one journal retyped in the style of another before they can resubmit it.

Otherwise, I have thoroughly revised *Better Medical Writing* in the light of what I have learnt in the last six years. In doing this, I hope I have not plagiarised the work of the many friends whose articles and books I have read and whose lectures and talks I have listened to. I have consciously tried to avoid stealing anybody else's ideas, but if I have done so unwittingly I apologise; perhaps the book should be dedicated to 'my friends pictured within'.

Finally, I should like to thank some of the many people who have been concerned in the writing courses: Dr Yrjö Collan, of Helsinki; Professor Salem Damluji and Professor Fahan Bakir, of Baghdad; Dr Isadeen Shikhara of Mosul; Dr Bertie Wood of Perth; Dr Eoin O'Brien and Dr Noel Reilly of Dublin; Dr Sadat Sabri of Kuwait; and Dr Bahman Joorabchi of Shiraz.

July 1976   Stephen Lock

Preface to First Edition

I suspect that a large part of the formal scientific literature is hardly ever read at all.

Maddox, J., *Lancet*, 1968, ii, 1071

'Have you published anything?' The question usually comes at that sticky point in the interview, after the chairman has read aloud most of the facts on your application form. The candidate who can reply 'a couple of things in the *Lancet*' is at once streets ahead. It does not matter much what the things were. Even if the application form asked for details, the betting is that no one will ask about them. They were published, and that is enough.

But, to be more serious, the primary purpose of most authors is, or should be, to advance knowledge—to communicate the results of their work to their colleagues and contemporaries. The trouble is that while appointments committees continue to demand lists of published work candidates will continue to provide them, irrespective of the quality of the contents or the style. Even in good academic units workers are often under some pressure to get a paper out before their grants are due to be renewed. Add to these pressures on most authors their lack of training in scientific method or in the rudiments of English style, and it is not surprising that the 15,000 medical manuscripts submitted for publication every year in Britain make depressing reading for the editors who receive them. Half the articles should never have been sent in, and of the 10 per cent that record good, original work no more than a handful are written in a style that makes for easy reading.

In a book of just under 100 pages nobody can produce a formula that will turn any doctor into a good scientific author overnight. What I hope to do, however, is to give guidance to inexperienced authors, particularly the registrar or senior registrar, who in a few years has to publish four or five papers, to move up a grade, to keep up with the Joneses, to enter in the *Medical Directory*, or for some such motive. Once he has obtained a consultant post, this doctor will write papers less often and with more pleasure. So the early sections of the book advise him on what to write about, how to set about it, and where to send it for publication.

Writing this book would have been unnecessary if registrars and others could be told that all they had to do was to look at the medical journal and follow the pattern of the articles in them. But, unfortunately, usually the hungry sheep would look up—and not be fed. Thus, the second, and more important, reason I had for writing about medical authorship was its present low standard. Even experienced authors too often seem to believe that serious work must be described in the curiously tortured obscure style often used at present, and lectures and teaching articles that should be models of clarity are often presented in this unintelligible way. I hope to show that even complicated subjects can be discussed in simple, clear English.

Whatever your reasons for writing an article, the process of writing it will have some beneficial effects. The first article is undoubtedly the most difficult of all. Whether or not this first attempt is published, as an author you will be forced to learn your way round a medical library and to become familiar with indexing and references. More important, however, you will also begin to learn the principles of scientific or clinical research, for publication should show up any defects in your approach and encourage you to put these right. At the same time, even the most trivial piece of research is likely to stimulate further questions to answer. One paper will lead to others.

Charles Thorne

1 *When to Start*

*For many doctors the achievement of a published article is a tedious duty
to be surmounted as a necessary hurdle in a medical career. You have got to
get over it, just as you have to dissect a dogfish for the first M.B.; you don't
like it, but it's got to be done. Though the subject of an article is important
it is not much to do with its dullness. I believe if a man has something to
say which interests him, and he knows how to say it, then he need never be
dull. Unfortunately some people have a desire for publication but nothing
more. They have nothing to say, and they do not know how to say it. They
want to be seen in the* British Medical Journal *or the* Lancet *because it is
respectable to be seen there, like being seen in a church.*

Asher, R., *British Medical Journal*, 1958, **2**, 502

Soon after qualification you may have realised that you will have
to publish some papers if you are not to be judged lazy, or stupid,
or both. First, however, get your priorities right. If your ambition
is to be a consultant in the hospital service, or to work in a university department, then for the two or three years of house appointments your main target should be the Membership or Fellowship.
The longer you spend in a specialty, the more difficult these
examinations become. Until they are out of the way, publication
should be considered only if by chance a ready-made paper comes
your way. You may be lucky, however, and be concerned in the
management of a patient with a rare condition or with an unusual
presentation of a common one. How should such cases be 'written
up'?

Case reports

Case reports fall into two classes: 'funnies' and 'heavies'. Funnies
are curiosities of clinical practice that have no implications for
other doctors who may meet similar cases. Bizarre foreign bodies
in curious sites—such as Hamilton Bailey's turnip in the rectum—
and world-record-size lipomata are examples. Such cases are

usually best reported in a short letter to a weekly journal or to the journal of the hospital or medical school. It is pointless for a busy houseman to spend a lot of effort searching reference books and writing up a long discussion of earlier cases of the same kind. Indeed, the chances of publication are reduced if the editor is reminded that, for example, nineteen cases of swallowed billiard balls have been recorded already.

Heavies are clinical or pathological rarities of scientific importance, and by recording the facts the author has added something of value. In recent years many important clinical syndromes have become recognised after several reports of single cases or small series. Examples are bird fancier's lung, some of the non-metastatic manifestations of bronchial carcinoma, and lactic acidosis. A heavy may still be presented as a simple letter: 'While doing a period as a locum tenens in a practice in Dorset I saw a case of nocardiosis in a 43-year-old housewife . . . ', in which the history, examination, and findings are presented as though on a ward round, Many of these letters may be included in the *Index Medicus*, so that they are not to be despised.

At the other extreme is the Rolls-Royce of case reports, the 600-word short report, which requires a lot of effort from the authors. You must find out how original the condition is. When was the first case reported? (Hippocrates? Avicenna? Heberden? Osler?) Where did the most recent case report appear (?*J. Nepal. med. Ass.*)? Who published the largest series reported in the last few years? Then you should decide if your case adds anything to those already published. If the condition has been reported several times before and lacks new features (such as response to a new drug when no specific treatment had been thought to exist) then the case is not original enough to make a short report. Solitary case reports rarely are, unless the author can find a new angle.

Effects of drugs

Reports of side-effects of drugs are frequently submitted to medical journals. The first thing the editor does is to check with the latest edition of the *Excerpta Medica* publication, *Side Effects of Drugs*. Every reported effect of all common drugs is listed, and, if there is more than one listing, the chances of a single report being published are very poor. Even if the report is original, it should be kept short; what matters is that the adverse effect should be recorded, so that others may look out for it. If it is serious, then any evidence supporting the link between drug and danger should be quoted. But, as with case reports, single-patient events rarely make more than letters.

New treatments for migraine, psoriasis, and asthma are constantly being discovered by doctors who want to report uncontrolled trials of five patients with an 80 per cent success rate. This might have been all right twenty years ago, but it is not any more, even as a letter. On the other hand, reports of patients poisoned by drugs and other toxic substances are valuable, especially if the treatment given was lifesaving. The effects of agricultural and industrial chemicals on man frequently come to light only after a series of accidental or suicidal poisonings. Very often the manufacturers can give information about earlier reports, and other good sources of information are your local poisons centre and the Committee on Safety of Medicines.

Collecting rare cases

Rare conditions are necessarily seen rarely, but an account of an unfamiliar condition is more reliable if based on several cases. An alternative to writing up the case at once is to present it at the appropriate section of the Royal Society of Medicine (R.S.M.) or at a meeting of a local medical society, when there is a fair chance that other clinicians will come forward with similar cases. A more authoritative paper can then be written by several authors together.

New appliances

Clinicians often devise small pieces of apparatus which help in a routine diagnostic procedure and some medical journals have a regular section for new appliances. Orthopaedic surgeons always seem to be inventing plates, screws, and splints, and if they can persuade a reputable manufacturer to make the apparatus they may also be able to persuade an editor to publish an account of it, though usually such reports are best sent to the journal in the relevant specialty.

3

Articles of this kind must be descriptions of truly new inventions, and you should be able to report that you have used them in patients with some success. You should keep this article as short as possible and send a selection of photographs and drawings so that the journal can make a choice.

Finally, at this stage in your career, keep an eye open for the chance of a letter to a weekly journal commenting on a paper or an article in an earlier issue. This subject is discussed in detail in a later chapter, but one piece of advice bears noting here. Submit nothing for publication without showing it to your chief—the professor if you are in an academic department, the consultant in a hospital. Often he will be able to make useful suggestions, and occasionally he will stop you making a fool of yourself. He is after all responsible for the standards of his unit, and it is misplaced kindness to think that by adding his name to the article you are doing him a favour. Nothing annoys a respected physician more easily than finding a stupid or conceited letter from his houseman in one of the weeklies.

2 'Research' or What Not to Write

Authors who write Original Articles really do not have a varied reader-ship in mind. To the contrary, they use concepts, language, symbolism, and methodologic descriptions that will attract and impress the co-expert. The reasons for this are obvious. Acceptability of the article for publication will be judged first by reviewers who are specialists, and then by similarly qualified and hypercritical readers. If the peer specialist happens to be a department chief or a man otherwise influential in the reaches of academic medicine, so much the better for the young author's status and his chances for advancement.

Ingelfinger, F. J., *Science*, 1970, **169**, 831

Really interesting cases are always worth recording, and many would argue that professional men have a duty to report them to their colleagues; but, after acquiring a higher degree, the would-be consultant has a special interest in publishing the results of some original research. Though clinical research is more glamorous, and may appeal to the practical doctor, it is much less certain to yield suitable material than rat work. A carefully designed laboratory study should be guaranteed to produce original results, and a good piece of research could easily provide material for an MD thesis, several papers published in conference proceedings, and two or three original articles in reputable journals.

A year or so as a junior lecturer, demonstrator, or research assistant is time well spent; whether or not every budding consultant benefits from a period of research, undoubtedly appointments committees are impressed by it. A junior member of a good unit has access to advice on suitable subjects to study and on techniques, and he may be able to do some dull but necessary work in a more elaborate research project, and so get his name on the paper. A chance of a junior appointment linked with a research unit should be seized before someone else steps in.

The value of such an appointment lies not in the specialised knowledge of, say, embryonic deformities induced by cyclamates, but in the training it gives in scientific method. All good articles

5

begin well before the actual research work with planning that implicates the statistician and the librarian, as well as thinking of the individual journal in which they may be published. Proper design of experiments, quality control, comparability of results—all these essentials for valid scientific investigation should be acquired as habits during a research assistantship.

Clinical research

Even so, most young doctors find themselves doing routine clinical work. Can they do research at the same time? The sad truth is that much so-called clinical research is futile for all concerned.

Faced with the prospect of two years' grind as a registrar in a diabetic clinic every Tuesday and Thursday afternoon, you may console yourself that at least you should get a paper out of it. You may—but you will have to be clever, and lucky. Too many clinicians in Britain spend years recording everything imaginable; for example, height, weight, age, sex, blood sugar, blood pressure, urine analysis, retinal appearances, ECG, and chest X-ray, from 500 diabetics (or hypertensives, or dyspeptics, or whatever) taking one or two established drugs. The findings of such a study are predictable. The work has all been done before. If the results confirm earlier studies, then there is no real point in saying so: if they differ from all earlier work, then very good reasons will be needed to convince the editor and his assessors that the results are reliable. Magpie collection of statistics for no better reason than the accumulation of 'raw data', followed by an aimless feeding of figures into a computer, produces nothing of value for writing up. Even so, there is something to be said for 'unoriginal' research done for one's own satisfaction or as a form of quality control of the unit's work; not uncommonly, senior academics carry on with this type of work long after their truly original ideas are spent, but they do not try to publish their results.

Many aspects of common disorders have yet to be investigated fully; in the last two years good papers have been published in leading journals on the management of appendicitis, perforated peptic ulcer, myocardial infarction, and pneumonia. Bear in mind, however, that usually only positive findings are of interest, though of course a 'positive' finding might include, for example, a report that there was no case of hypertension among 1,000

6

consecutive primiparous Carib Indians. It is sad that there is no *Journal of Negative Results*; perhaps one day a philanthropist will start one.

As a registrar with a diabetic clinic to run you must, if you want to do useful research, study journals such as *Diabetes*, attend meetings, talk to senior colleagues, ask questions, get advice. In this way you should look for a question that is worth answering. What you should look for particularly is a comment in a paper from a good unit that some findings need confirmation, or that it is not known whether the serum concentration of some enzyme is the same in diabetics as in normal people. You may find a report in a foreign journal (including those published in the U.S.A.) of a 'first', in which case the first report in Britain should be worth recording in a British journal. Another aspect is the local pattern of disease. It is important that each individual medical community should know whether the incidence and prevalence of common illnesses are the same as those classically described for the Western world. Publishing these is the ideal role for the local medical journal, for rarely are the findings of widespread interest. On the other hand, just because a question is unanswered does not necessarily mean that it deserves an answer; for example, correlations of fluoride content of hair with the blood sugar is of trivial importance unless it can be shown to be of clinical importance.

Investigations should be kept as simple as possible, but studies of biochemical value in groups of patients must be properly constructed so that the results are scientifically reliable. This usually means that the correct control group must be studied, and a statistician's advice is invaluable here, and that the right ethical decisions are taken before you start the work. Occasionally, original work of scientific interest is turned down by a good journal on the grounds that the study was unethical (*see* Appendix D).

Drug trials

The search for a suitable question to answer can be disheartening, especially if two or three good ideas have to be discarded because preliminary screening of published papers shows that the work has already been done. In these circumstances there is a grave temptation to do a drug trial. Poor trials are easy; good ones are time-consuming and difficult to arrange. Most promising new drugs are given their first clinical trials in medical units with established reputations. A top-class drug house will not make samples of a new drug available to an unknown junior physician in an undistinguished hospital. So the clinician with no established reputation has two possibilities open to him: he may try out an established drug in the treatment of a condition for which it has not been used before, or he may conduct a trial of a new product from a smaller drug house. In either case a small pilot study is essential: negative results are hardly ever worth publishing.

If the pilot study suggests that the trial is likely to give positive results, then speed is important. It is common experience that trials of a new treatment are done in several centres at the same time. The first two or three papers on the subject will find much readier acceptance than the others. Authors still write to medical journals saying, 'as you recently published two papers on the use of manganese citrate in the treatment of ulcerative colitis I am sending you my report of thirty-two patients treated with high doses of manganese for twelve months', and wonder why the paper is swiftly returned. In this field more than any other there is no justice. A perfectly designed and scrupulously performed double-blind crossover study is of negligible interest if two or three sound but less polished papers have already appeared. On the other hand, the time when an uncontrolled trial of a drug could be published has now passed, with the rare exception of a preliminary communication about the first use of a really new drug.

It is a waste of time to repeat trials that have been done before unless new findings can be reported. Just as useless are trials of drugs having no advantage over their competitors. 'New' anti-biotic derivatives come on the market in a steady stream, and their makers claim that they make the established compounds out of date. Verifying such claims needs long, large-scale trials, with careful statistical planning and comparison with existing agents of proved value, and research of this kind is beyond the scope of most unestablished clinical investigators. Similarly, trials of well-known treatments are not to be undertaken lightly. A neurologist may believe that corticotrophin has no therapeutic action in ex-acerbations of multiple sclerosis. Any further trials on this subject will need to be beyond reproach on scientific grounds if they are to be published, and it may well be that no controlled trial is

8

possible since it would be considered unethical to withhold treatment from any patients.

Anybody undertaking a drug trial should consult the standard article by N. D. W. Lionel and A. Herxheimer (*British Medical Journal*, 1970, **3**, 637), which gives a detailed check list of all the items that should be considered. This emphasises that a third of the articles that they analysed were considered unacceptable because of inadequate or inappropriate methods; controls not used when required or inadequate; or statistics not reported when required. As an example they cite a trial of an antihypertensive drug, carried out by 38 GPs: 'The report described the method used in one sentence: "Blood pressure readings were taken before and after a period of treatment not less than 12 weeks and not exceeding 16 weeks." Such use of casual and unstandardised measurements is inadequate for assessing drug effects on blood pressure.'

Inevitable rejections

Editors are often asked how they select an article for publication from the vast number of papers submitted to them. Authors are usually surprised that editors do not find it all that difficult. Half the papers can be rejected after no more than a few minutes' study. These inevitable rejections fall into three classes.

Review articles bringing important subjects up to date are commissioned by editors. If a doctor feels that his experience qualifies him to write such an article, he should first ask the editor of the journal of his choice: he may be lucky, and if so he will be told for what type of reader it should be written, how long to make it, how many illustrations to include, how many references, and so on. But the clinical features, pathological findings, and management of carcinoma of the body of the pancreas are adequately described in several contemporary textbooks, and an enthusiastic registrar is unlikely to do it better.

Hypotheses often fall into the same class as review articles. Most of those published by good journals have been commissioned from a leading authority in the subject, or at the very least the author consulted the editor before submitting the article. If you believe strongly that your idea is sound, then the logical conclusion is to find some data that support it, or try to prove it by a well-designed experiment. If the facilities are not available to you then you must persuade someone who has them to do the work for you.

Retrospective surveys are almost invariably unsuccessful. Sifting through the case-notes of all patients with renal colic admitted to a particular unit in a five-year period is unlikely to turn up anything of value. The records cannot be expected to be complete, and the only way to find out whether or not the patients had eaten pork in the twenty-four hours preceding the onset of abdominal pain is to do a prospective trial and to spend five years asking them.

Regular publication

Once you have published your first dozen papers, you will have established a reputation in your specialty. This has two implications: first, editors will be more inclined to publish your papers with less scrutiny than those written by unknown authors, and, secondly, you no longer need to publish as often as possible.

This means you must impose a strict self-censorship. Before settling down to write another article, examine your motives. Have you really something important to add to knowledge on the subject? Scores of workers in other countries will send out automatic reprint requests, but they will soon tire of reading your papers if the effort is not rewarded by new knowledge. Moreover, an editor soon realises when a previous authority is producing second-rate work, and probably over-reacts against him. No matter how sound your reputation, you can lose it by ill-considered publication of trivial papers that add nothing to your earlier work.

Do not be tempted by the modern trend of releasing results in driblets. If you set about a three-year study of the effects of surgical treatment of lichen planus, then wait until you have the results before publishing them. Too often one sees a study of this kind presented as a preliminary communication (six cases, showing encouraging results), at mid-point (twenty-nine cases, average follow-up ten months), and again at the end—the time that had been already selected when the results would have statistical validity.

Finally, do not let your name appear on a paper unless you are completely happy about the work. Your collaborators in a trial that failed to show significant results may insist on submitting an article. If you believe the work was not worth recording, then withdraw from being an author, but politely. Having done so, keep quiet about it.

As a senior man in a unit, you may be following tradition by appearing among the authors of all papers from it. If so, then you must read them all if sooner or later you are not to be embarrassed.

There is no hard and fast rule about the order in which authors' names should appear. Some units use the alphabetical system; in others the senior's name always comes last. Until there is some agreed rule, there is a good case for starting with the man who had the idea or did the work; in this way every member of a unit should appear as a first author at some time in his career. Some have also argued that, with the principal in front, and the chief at the end, the authors in the middle should be placed in descending order according to the importance of their contribution to the work. However theoretically ideal such a system, I can foresee nothing but bickering and wasted time resulting from it, and believe that there is much to be said for putting middle authors in alphabetical order.

3 *When You have Decided*

For most doctors, writing a paper is a fairly important step in their professional lives. It should therefore be treated like other important steps. Do you remember when you were deciding which job to apply for, which specialty to choose, which house to buy? You did not plunge into any of these without any thought at all; instead, you read round the subject, and asked other people, whether connected with the subject or outside it. Only then did you make up your mind. Much the same care should be taken before writing a series of case reports, or doing work in a laboratory, or starting a survey, and the problem should be approached as methodically as possible.

The search for information

The first question anybody outside the project will ask is, 'What has been done before?', and it will be no good seeking expert advice unless you know this. To give you a few references, start with some papers that have already covered an aspect of the work in question. Good sources of information are leading articles in journals, review articles of the kind published in the *British Journal of Hospital Medicine*, and the exhaustive articles, part-original/part-review, that appear in the *Quarterly Journal of Medicine (Baltimore)*. *Current Contents* is a valuable collection of the contents pages of most important journals, and will give you an idea of what recent articles have been appearing in your specialty. After this, consult the *Index Medicus* of the last four or five years to fill in the gaps. Today most medical libraries take the *Index*; if you are not already familiar with it, first read the subject headings (printed in the January issue every year) so that you miss nothing because of the inevitable quirks of classification. The list of review articles published in the *Index* every month may be a short cut to getting references on your subject, while books such as the *Yearbook* and *Progress In* series and the *Medical Annual* may be used as a final check that you have missed no important original work on the subject.

Next approach your librarian for advice, showing him what you have found out already. Treat him as the specialist he is, and you will be well rewarded. He may be able to produce a few more key references for you and will certainly get you copies of the articles you need, either in the actual journals or as photostats, which can nowadays be got cheaply from the R.S.M. or the B.M.A. He can also arrange to get from the National Lending Library photostats of articles published in unusual journals. The National Library of Medicine in the U.S.A. also has a computer system of information retrieval, based on the *Index Medicus*, known as Medlars. All articles listed in *Index Medicus* are entered into the computer's magnetic-tape memory bank, and a research worker who wants a list of all published work about a topic can arrange for a 'search' to be made. The computer then prints out all the articles of any relevance—usually an enormous list, most of which can be discarded at once. Medlars searches are expensive, but it is often worth asking the librarian whether one has already been made on your subject; if it has, he should be able to arrange for you to see a copy. Another source of searches is the library at the R.S.M., which keeps lists of references obtained previously for Fellows of the Society.

All this sounds as if it might take days of work, but it will probably need only two or three hours in a library. The recent rapid growth of medical libraries in postgraduate centres throughout the country means that now even the isolated doctor has access to the books and journals he needs. But to keep up with all these references it is a good idea to write each one down in full on a separate filing card: this should give all the authors and their initials, the title of the article in full, the name of the journal in full, the year, volume number, and first and last pages of the article.

You now know what has been done before, which questions remain unanswered, and those points on which other workers have disagreed. The time has come to discuss the paper or the underlying work with your colleagues. Do not be afraid that they will want to get their names on the paper or to do the same work more quickly on the sly. Most of them will have written papers when they were younger, and you can learn a lot from their mistakes. Also, quite often, somebody may be able to tell you about another man who is doing, or is about to publish, similar work, or who can put you in touch with an expert on the subject. Even if your subject is really original, advice from colleagues is still always worth while, for they may be able to suggest short cuts or indicate the snags in a particular approach. Before you consult them, however, you should have a good idea of what you are aiming at: a thesis, fulllength original article (perhaps the first of a series), case report, review article, a presentation at a conference.

If the paper deals with a new drug, quite possibly you have already been in touch with the medical adviser of the company concerned; if not, do contact him. He may know of similar work going on elsewhere, with which you might combine to produce a joint paper of much greater authority. Incidentally, you may also find that drug houses may be able to help you in other ways. If the laboratory work needed is complex, they might help you by doing this themselves, or by lending you the equipment and an assistant. They may also help with incidental expenses for your work or even provide you with funds to attend conferences on the subject. Usually, there is nothing unprofessional about this, for most firms realise that it is not in their real interests to bribe or influence you in any way.

Once the subject of the paper and its probable destination have been decided, find a statistician at the planning stage before you do any work that brings in figures. It is no good doing the work and then presenting a statistician with a mass of figures and asking him to work out P and χ^2 if the results are not capable of valid analysis. You should understand how the statistician treats your data, otherwise you will not be able to write the paper clearly, so read a book about statistics, such as the excellent one by Bradford Hill (*see* Appendix E, p. 114).

Similarly, if your work deals with population studies and entails surveys or questionnaires, first get the help of an epidemiologist. It is tragic how many papers editors have to reject because their authors have compared different population groups or obtained results over different periods of time, or have used questionnaires that have not been validated. Unless you can show good reasons for excluding a factor, comparable populations must have the same distribution of subjects classified by race, sex, age, weight, occupation, social class, and environment. In retrospective surveys the research often shows that one group of patients had surgical treatment and another medical, and that the groups differ when analysed on factors that were relevant to the decision of whether or not to operate. If an advance is made in medical or surgical treatment of the condition, neither group will be comparable for any future study. Once again, if possible, expert advice should be sought before the research is done. A good book to read about this is Witt's *Clinical Trials* (*see* Appendix E).

In any paper that reports experimental work most editors are now very pernickety about the ethical aspects—and rightly so. 'Informed consent', after the procedure has been fully explained to the patient or his relatives, or both, should always be obtained (and the fact specifically mentioned in the text of the article, together with whether some patients refused to take part and whether the work is as approved by an ethical committee). Ethical principles are discussed in greater detail in Appendix D on p. 111 but if you are still in any doubt whether the work is ethical or not you should do two things: ask yourself whether you would mind the same procedure being carried out on any of your relatives, and discuss the ethical aspects with as many colleagues as possible, including the hospital ethical committee, if one exists.

4 Where to Send Your Article

True there is competition but the traditional medical journal still has the support of the bulk of the medical profession They stand up to the critical issue of their printed word being read.

New Zealand Medical Journal, 1975, **81**, 307

Before you start writing your article you should have a good idea of the journal in which you want to publish your article. Apart from the medical newspapers and drug-company handouts there are three main types of journal—general, specialist (which includes college, society, and local publications), and review. How do you decide which one to aim at?

General journals have the advantages of a large, international, audience and quick publication. Their obvious disadvantage is the high rejection rate of about 85 per cent. The reason for this is not that editors are harsh (in fact most of them hate saying 'no'), but because they cannot publish more than a limited number of articles every week without boring their readers or going bankrupt. A rough balance sheet (for the *B.M.J.*, anyway) might work out as follows:

	Submitted %	Accepted %
Outstanding original work	5	5
Crazy, unsupported speculations	2	0
Unsuited to particular journal (too specialised, not in appropriate field, etc.)	45	0
Unoriginal, poor scientific quality, inadequate statistics, unethical	29	0
Remaining for decision	19	10

So every editor, but especially the editor of a general journal (whose readers rely on him to certify that an article outside their own specialty is sound) must ask several questions about every article submitted. Is it original (for the world or for the country)? If not, is its importance sufficient to outweigh this objection; for example, does it emphasise a danger not sufficiently appreciated? Are the scientific views sound, the ethics beyond reproach, and the statistics valid? Will the article really interest the non-specialist reader?

All these features influence an editor one way or the other. You can also sometimes tip the balance in your favour by presenting the article itself in the best possible way—a subject discussed in the next two chapters. This kind of routine makes life much easier for the editor of a general journal, and it should also help you as an author to know whether it is worth submitting an article or not.

The Lancet

There are two main general journals in Britain, the *British Medical Journal* and the *Lancet*. The older of the two, the *Lancet*, has a circulation of about 50,000 (roughly one-third in Britain, one-third in the U.S.A., and one-third elsewhere). If one can classify such things, it is the more 'left-wing' of the two, with racy and hard-hitting editorials, and good international coverage; it is also read by many more people than those who subscribe to it. Because, usually, they do not believe in refereeing articles, the editors usually let you know very quickly whether they want to publish your article or not, and after acceptance they publish it within a few weeks. Very often, however, even if they do accept your article they will ask you to shorten it, and when you get the galley proofs you may find that it has been styled in *Lancet* prose, which manages to make your points much clearer than you ever thought possible (though it is fair to say that not all authors like this styling). The *Lancet* also has a section for 'middle articles', which covers a wide variety of subjects, while many scientific findings may be published as long letters to the Editor.

The *Lancet* has developed two tendencies in recent years. Firstly, many of the original articles now come from outside Britain, particularly from the U.S.A. and Scandinavia. The second tendency has been towards publication of very preliminary work, often in animals, with potential clinical implications. This means that if you have some tentative, but exciting and potentially important experimental work in animals, which you want to put to a wide audience at an early stage, the *Lancet* probably is your best bet for a first try. But do not be disappointed if they cannot help you.

British Medical Journal (B.M.J.)

While it is obviously impossible to place journals in water-tight compartments, the *B.M.J.* is still firmly rooted in clinical medicine. This is not to say that its articles are not original or highbrow —they are both—but most of them have fairly obvious, and immediate, application to the patient. The circulation is about 85,000, the largest for a medical journal outside the U.S.A., and 20,000 of these copies go abroad, so that, with the 20 per cent or so of articles the *B.M.J.* publishes from abroad, again the international coverage is good. Though the journal is owned by the B.M.A., its policy concerning the original articles is entirely independent.

As well as a section for original articles, which includes Short Reports (limited to 600 words, 5 references, and 1 table or figure) and Side Effects, it also contains a Medical Practice Section, which includes unsolicited Review Articles and papers on the organisation of medical care, and the *Supplement*, which may print Talking Points—articles on medicopolitical topics. Few articles are accepted unmodified; usually, the authors are asked to shorten them and possibly also, on the referee's advice, to add or alter certain passages. Once accepted, articles may also be slightly changed in subediting. Because it is committed to refereeing almost any article potentially suitable for publication, the *B.M.J.* takes a little longer than the *Lancet* to decide whether to accept your article and in actually publishing it. Usually, if the *B.M.J.* rejects your article it does not send a referee's report back with it, though one is often available on request. Articles are often rejected not for their poor scientific quality but because they are quite unsuitable for that journal as regards subject matter or treatment. Authors of long articles that cannot be shortened (either because excision would leave out really important matter, or because the author is unwilling to have this done) often cannot understand that to publish an article that occupies a quarter or a third of the entire contents of the journal is just not feasible.

By and large, if you have some truly original work concerned more or less directly with human disease and your account is fairly brief and you do not want it abbreviated very much, I would advise you to try the *B.M.J.*

Do not be surprised, however, if the editor of either the *Lancet* or the *B.M.J.* regrets, etc., and suggests a specialist journal. Whatever you may think, he is as interested in publishing new, exciting, and important work as you are, and he also has a much better idea than you have of what his readers want (or ought to want). There is also a fair chance if your work is really good and printed in a specialist journal that it will be picked up by the general journals and discussed in a leader. In this way you may get at least two mentions for one article.

Other general journals

In Britain there are several other general journals. The *Scottish Medical Journal* contains articles, lectures, and accounts of meetings, mostly with a Scottish flavour. The *Postgraduate Medical Journal* is an ideal journal in which to try to place a well-written piece, of general interest, that does not report original findings. The *Quarterly Journal of Medicine* contains a mixture of original and review articles and is considered on p. 21. Elsewhere, most other national medical associations have their own journals, the *Journal of the American Medical Association* (*J.A.M.A.*) having the largest circulation of any medical journal in the world. Most of these, whether from policy or merely from practice, seem to confine themselves to publishing work from their own countries, and unless one has worked in a team, say, in the States or in Australia, there is not much point in trying them if your article has already been rejected by the *B.M.J.* or the *Lancet*, or both.

One journal, the *New England Journal of Medicine*, sometimes does publish work from outside the States. Though it may lack the breadth of the *Lancet*'s originals, the zest of the *B.M.J.*'s correspondence, and the wide coverage of *J.A.M.A.*, its printing and layout are superb, the medical intelligence always worth reading, and almost all the original articles important. In a subprofession not known for its compliments there are few medical journalists who do not admire and actually praise this journal. But before you are tempted too much, remember that it publishes only three or four originals every week and that there is often an obvious special reason why a particular paper from outside the States has been accepted.

Specialist journals

By now it will be obvious to you that most doctors will have to publish most of their articles in specialist journals. Apart from the subject matter of the articles they print, specialist journals differ little from general ones. Do not imagine therefore that you can get away with a lower standard of scientific, ethical, or statistical reliability in a specialist journal. You will find that the editor has definite criteria of his own, and in any case his rejection rate will still be 40 to 50 per cent. A specialist journal editor is less concerned about the degree of originality and the remoteness of the subject from a general medical reader with little knowledge of the specialty. Thus, he is likely to look favourably on a largish series of patients with a rare disease studied with all the latest techniques, and he may well accept single case-reports of ultra-rare conditions that are useful reminders for workers in the particular specialty.

Almost all specialties now have their own journals in Britain, America, and Scandinavia, and often there are several covering only particular aspects of the subject, such as the *Journal of Neurochemistry*. How do you choose which specialist journal you should send your article to? Possibly you belong to a specialist society that has a journal of its own, usually publishing articles of broad general interest. Try this journal if you think your article would be suitable, but choose a more specialised one if your subject is esoteric for doctors even within the specialty. It does not matter if this latter journal is not published in your own country, for it is better to get an informed audience of experts than one who will not appreciate your work. For example, many articles on blood diseases might well be submitted first to the *British Journal of Haematology*, or the *Journal of Clinical Pathology*, but one on the more rarefied laboratory aspects of coagulation would often better be sent straight away to a journal such as *Thrombosis et Diathesis Haemorrhagica*, published in Germany, which contains papers in English, German, and French.

The pecking order of your choice of journals will depend on you and the nature of your article. While you have been preparing this, and consulting references, you will have had a good chance to assess the standards of such journals and to find out what sort of articles they accept. Remember also that many journals cut across specialties, so that, for instance, a paper on Reiter's disease could be submitted to an ophthalmological, venereological, or rheumatological journal, and in some cases to one devoted to social medicine or medical illustration.

Finally, delays in publication with specialist journals are usually much longer than with general journals, often varying from six to eighteen months. This is not really as bad as it sounds. Once your article has been accepted you can give the journal as a reference 'in the press', and many journals will give you correct priority by stating the date they received your article.

Review journals

Under this heading I am including two types of journal—those that publish review articles proper and a few original articles or case reports, and those that publish articles which are both a 'review of the literature' and a report of a series of personally studied patients. The prototype of the first category is the *Practitioner*, and in Britain there are also the *British Journal of Hospital Medicine* and *Update*. The primary aim of these journals is instruction, either as a refresher course or to help a candidate preparing for a higher examination. Though this type of journal may accept a few proffered articles, most of the articles are commissioned for a particular issue with a particular view-point in mind. So it is a good idea to ask the editor of a journal of this kind whether he would like to see your article (which you should briefly describe) before you send it to him.

The second type of review journal is typified by the *Quarterly Journal of Medicine, Medicine (Baltimore)*, the *American Journal of Medicine*, and the *Annals* and *Archives of Internal Medicine*. The character of all of these, particularly the first three, differs considerably from the other types of journal, in that an author is usually given enough space to present his findings in the perspective of earlier ones. The total length is usually greater than that allowed in most other journals; the introduction is often long, with an extensive survey of previous work; case histories are given in detail, and often extended tables and figures are used;

and the discussion is considered under several separate headings. Hence these articles are frequently the standard reference on a particular topic for several years. To be accepted, therefore, an article of this type must deal either with many patients with a fairly common disease studied from a particular aspect, or with a few with a rare condition studied intensively. This is the one occasion where a thesis really comes into its own, for it satisfies most of the requirements. But be careful. Beware of just sending off the separate pages of the thesis, perhaps joined together with some connecting phrases, for almost always it will be unsuitable. Rewrite the material entirely as a new article. This is a great deal of work, but if your article is accepted it is well worth while because an article of this kind carries immense prestige.

5 Choosing Among Some American Journals

GEORGE DUNEA

Thus in practical activities the American love for novelty and their lack of circumspection has led to great achievements which are too well known to call for enumeration. In contrast, dire results have ensued from the operation of the same bias in domains where there are no immanent mechanisms for eliminating error: where correctness and falsehood are normally a matter of degree, and truth can only be partially gleaned by a laborious crawl over dangerous ground between attractively camouflaged traps, and where every step calls for a suspicious examination and often a suspended judgment; and to top it all, where excessive incredulity can be just as misleading as gullibility.

Andreski, Stanslav, *Social Sciences as Sorcery,*
André Deutsch, London, 1972

The secret to successful writing, in America as in England, is to have something to say, to say it well, to follow the principles of scientific composition, and to choose the right journal for your manuscript. Research papers, results of drugs trials, and clinical reports on a series of patients constitute the bread and butter of medical journalism, general reviews serve a useful purpose, but single case reports are less popular with editors, especially when used as excuse for an exhaustive review of 'the literature'.

It is not absolutely necessary to use the American way of spelling when submitting papers to North American journals, yet an attempt to do so might earn the gratitude of harassed editors and proof-readers, as might the use of the American generic term for those drugs where the British name is not the same (for example, frusemide *vs* furosemide, pethidine *vs* meperidine). Virtually all American journals have their manuscripts reviewed by consultants who are experts in the subject of the paper. This increases the time for decision, but offers the author frequently useful criticism and suggestions for revision. The consultants' criticisms may or may not be returned with rejected manuscripts, depending on the journal.

General journals

In the United States, a blurred line divides general journals from those directed at the specialist internist, so that these periodicals are best considered together. Most of them enjoy a wide readership and a well-deserved popularity. Manuscript rejection rates are high, somewhere between 70 and 90 per cent, but these figures are distorted by the submission of many clearly unsuitable manuscripts. Generally, they make a decision within two months, but sometimes longer, and the publication time after acceptance is usually about six months but is variable. The most widely circulated is the *Journal of the American Medical Association*, with a circulation rate of over one quarter of a million, and with papers that are clinical rather than research orientated. The journal's policy is to cater to the thousands of physicians in practice—often in small towns—rather than to the academicians, investigators, and specialists, who have their own journals. Thus, the journal aims to be first choice for the generalist and second choice for the specialist, and it includes in every issue several brief case-reports and clinical notes.

New England Journal of Medicine, published continuously since 1812, is the official journal of the Massachussets Medical Society. With 160,000 subscribers, it enjoys a high reputation for the excellent quality of its original contributions, reviews, and editorials, and currently ranks as the most prestigious journal in internal medicine. It is, nevertheless, a general journal, and you may find in it papers pertaining to surgery, orthopaedics, public health, paediatrics, genetics, and basic sciences. Directed mainly at a clinical audience, even the most specialised article is likely to have some general interest. The aim is to be general rather than narrow, and if your paper is too narrow in conceptual or practical appeal, you will be advised to send it to a specialist journal. Another prestigious journal is the *Annals of Internal Medicine*, published monthly by the American College of Physicians. It has about 75,000 subscribers, is directed mainly at the general internist and the specialised internist who wishes to have a broad view of internal medicine, and it invites the submisson of papers on clinical, laboratory, socioeconomic, cultural, and historical topics pertinent to internal medicine and related fields. Case reports may be presented as brief communications (1,500 words) or as letters (750 words). The *Archives of Internal Medicine*, is published monthly by the American Medical Association and has recently come under a new editorship. It has a circulation rate of 62,000, and is directed at the general internist, the subspecialist, and the more sophisticated general practitioner. Subspecialty orientated papers should, however, be also of general interest. Well-written case reports are considered. The publication delay, however, has been rather long, as is also the case with the *American Journal of Medicine* which, with a circulation rate of 33,000, enjoys a high and well-deserved reputation. Founded by the late Alexander Gutman, the 'green journal' publishes clinical studies and has long specialised in the presentation of 'well-studied cases'. Also highly regarded is *Medicine*, which is published every two months, has a lower circulation (5,600) and specialises in lengthy reviews of syndromes and diseases. Other journals include the *American Journal of Medical Sciences*, a less widely read journal which covers all aspects of internal medicine, and the *Journal of Chronic Diseases*, a general journal devoted to articles on various aspects of chronic illness. Several state medical journals cater to an even more limited audience, as do the local, county, or city medical society publications. Many hospitals and medical schools have their own journals, and some of these such as the *Mayo Clinic Proceedings*, the *Mount Sinai Journal of Medicine*, the *Cleveland Clinic Quarterly*, and the *Johns Hopkins Medical Journal* are well known and occasionally accept contributions from outsiders.

Specialist journals

Although specialists often publish in generalist journals, they also have journals of their own. These differ in prestige, subject matter, and editorial policies. Subjects range widely, from anaesthesia to law, education, mental deficiency, industrial hygiene, veterinary science, hypnosis, behavioural sciences, deafness, vision, sexuality, drug information, and speech therapy. Cardiologists most frequently publish in *Circulation*, the journal of the American Heart

Association, which tends to emphasise research and observations based on larger series of patients, or in the *American Journal of Cardiology*, the official publication of the American College of Cardiology, which is somewhat more clinically orientated and will publish a limited number of case reports. The *American Heart Journal* is also widely read by clinicians and includes some case reports, but has a publication lag that may exceed one year; another cardiology journal, *Circulation Research*, is devoted entirely to basic research; while *Chest* publishes both cardiological and pulmonary material, including a good number of case reports. The most popular journal of pulmonary medicine is the *American Review of Respiratory Disease*, the official bulletin of the American Thoracic Society. Formerly restricted to tuberculosis, it now covers clinical and research aspects of all forms of respiratory diseases. Many papers dealing with respiratory physiology are also published in the appropriate section of the *Journal of Applied Physiology*.

Gastroenterology, the prestigious 'blue journal', invites papers concerning all aspects of the digestive tract and liver, and is dedicated about two-thirds to research; while the *American Journal of Digestive Diseases*, the *American Journal of Gastroenterology*, and *Gastrointestinal Endoscopy* also publish research papers but are more clinically orientated. Nephrology papers may be submitted to *Kidney International*, the organ of the International Society of Nephrology, whose editorial offices are located in the United States; the *Transactions of the American Society for Artificial Organs* publish dialysis and transplantation work presented by members (or non-members by introduction) at its spring meeting; and *Transplantation* is concerned mainly with immunology but also accepts clinical papers.

Rheumatologists publish in *Arthritis and Rheumatism*; while the *Journal of Infectious Diseases* provides a forum for laboratory and clinical aspects of infectious diseases, medical microbiology, and immunology. Other periodicals cover the fields of epidemiology, public health, and tropical medicine, and also genetics, dermatology, and allergy. *Blood*, the official journal of the American Society of Hematology, has a wide spectrum of investigational and clinical haematological material; while more specialised material may be submitted to *Cancer*, *Transfusion*, or even the *American Journal of Clinical Pathology*. The *Journal of Clinical Endocrinology and Metabolism* is the most prestigious endocrinological journal, and covers both clinical medicine and basic sciences; *Metabolism*, and *Endocrinology*, however, publish largely research papers; while *Diabetes* has both clinical and investigational material. The *Archives of Neurology* and *Neurology* are the two main neurological journals; and other journals cover more specialised areas such as headache, electroencephalography, neurophysiology, and, of course, psychiatry.

Of the various surgical journals, the *Annals of Surgery* and *Surgery, Gynecology, and Obstetrics* tend to be more research orientated; while somewhat more clinical manuscripts are published in *Surgery*, the *American Journal of Surgery*, and the *Archives of Surgery*, the last being published by the American Medical Association and having a circulation of about 45,000. In addition, the *Journal of Surgical Research* publishes basic or clinical research surgical papers. Other journals cover subspecialties such as urology, orthopaedics, plastic surgery, or neurosurgery; eye, ear, nose, and throat; or obstetrics and gynaecology. The last includes *Surgery, Gynecology, and Obstetrics*, the *American Journal of Obstetrics and Gynecology*, and *Obstetrics and Gynecology*. The main journal dealing with diseases of childhood are *Pediatrics*, published by the American Academy of Pediatrics and mainly research orientated; the *Journal of Pediatrics*, more clinical; the *American Journal of Diseases of Childhood*, which publishes original articles as well as case reports; and *Clinical Pediatrics*, which is practical, emphasises management of clinical problems and is mainly directed at practising paediatricians. At the other extreme of age, at least four journals deal with clinical, investigative, or social aspects of ageing and geriatrics.

The *Journal of Clinical Investigations* and the *Journal of Laboratory and Clinical Medicine* are two prestigious basic research and experimental medical journals that consider suitable contributions from all fields of medicine. The former is the organ of the American Society for Clinical Investigation and represents the pinnacle of achievement for the young investigator. The *American Journal of Physiology* and the *Journal of Applied Physiology* are published by the American Society of Physiology and require authors to state in their transmittal letter the preferred subsection for their manuscript; papers are then numbered accordingly in the table of contents. The *Journal of Immunology* is the official publication of the American Association of Immunologists; and the *Journal of Experimental Medicine* is also heavily biased toward immunology. The *American Journal of Pathology* is the most scientific and experimental of the pathology journals, about 80 per cent of its material being devoted to animal work. The *Archives of Pathology* are more clinical, and will accept occasional case reports, as will the *American Journal of Clinical Pathology*, a practical journal dedicated to clinical pathology, morphology, chemistry, and new methods, and also reports of series or individual cases. *Laboratory Investigation*, the official organ of the International Pathological Society, is heavily biased towards experimental work.

In addition to journals, the many specialty societies invite submission of abstracts for their regular meetings, and these are an additional medium of preliminary publication. Non-members usually require an introduction from a member of the society. The policies of the societies vary: some will publish all submitted abstracts, others only a selected few, while in yet others an abstract accepted for presentation at a meeting is automatically published in a journal or in the transactions.

Where to send your manuscript

Clearly America offers a bewildering array of medical journals. Yet the decision where to send your manuscript may be difficult: the choice is not necessarily wide, the number of prestigious general journals is small, and even within specialties the selection is relatively limited. Moreover, the rejection rate among the first-class American journals runs close to 90 per cent; and many papers are rejected at first submission because they are sent to the wrong journal. In making a decision, you may derive some help by picking the brains of someone experienced in medical publishing, or by consulting American or Canadian friends; and you should take time to review past issues of your journal of choice before making a final decision. Some journals specialise exclusively in clinical or experimental topics, others have a particular style of their own, and conformity with the general subject matter and format of the journal will increase your chances of success. Several reference books are also available for consultation: Deaton's *Markets for Medical Authors* is somewhat out of date, but helpful because it lists the journals according to their specialty, and, being all inclusive, will refer to the multitude of periodicals which for obvious reasons could not be mentioned in this chapter.

The *Directory of Publishing Opportunities* provides detailed address information, circulation rates, frequency of publication, and manuscript information, as well as the average time required for an editorial decision and for publication of accepted manuscripts. The Magazine Section of *Literary Market Place* may also be found to contain useful information.

Perhaps the greatest difficulty for the inexperienced writer arises with the single case report. Unless the presented material serves to delineate a new syndrome, or usefully expand the knowledge of a well-known clinical condition, it is not likely to appeal to the editorial boards of the major general or specialist journals. At that stage you may decide to send your manuscript to a journal of more limited prestige and circulation; or you may choose to follow the ancients' precept and lock it up for nine years, which should allow ample time for second thoughts about the worth and significance of your contribution.

6 Who Cares About Style?

Science has never been successfully integrated into the life of society, mainly because too many scientists have for too long given the impression that they hold a privileged position as members of an elite who are accountable to no one but themselves. The writer who shrouds his language in expressions that sound erudite, mysterious and complex, only perpetuates this notion.

Kuehn, C., *Journal of the American Medical Association*, 1973, **226,** 452

Scientific writers are rarely literate. If a colleague tells a scientist that his latest article is difficult to understand, the writer is more likely to assume that his colleague is unintelligent than that his article is unintelligible. Such writers believe that discussions about style, choice of words, length of sentences, active and passive voices, subjunctives, and the like, are for non-scientific second-rate minds with nothing original to say, and are irrelevant for serious scientific workers. Unfortunately, this argument can be supported by reference to published accounts of important work, many of which are badly written. No editor will reject first-class research because it is in poor English, and few journals have enough staff to rewrite all the articles they publish. So why does style matter?

Simplicity and clarity are the features of good scientific writing. Nobody is asking you to write great literature, but your meaning must be readily understood. Good points to remember are that doctors not working in the subject should be able to understand the article, and so should a doctor whose native language is not English. Clarity also helps the editor and his advisers to assess the article, and almost certainly prejudices them in its favour. Clear thought can be expressed clearly; and a man with something of value to say has no need to pad out his account. Watson and Crick's account of the double-helix structure of DNA was communicated as a 900-word letter to *Nature*.

Badly written, obscure, over-long articles bore editors (who are likely to reject them) and bore their readers (who are unlikely to finish them). They take up valuable space in journals, and they waste the time of the small group of readers for whom they are obligatory reading. In other words, most writers are failing to communicate—the object of writing in the first place.

In any article there are five critical features which, consciously or unconsciously, will influence an uncommitted reader to read the article and the editor to accept it for publication. These are: the total length of the article, the title, the introducion, the first few sentences of the discussion, and the summary.

Length of the article

The importance of keeping an article short is obvious, but it is surprising how everybody will agree yet not apply it to their own articles. Few people will read more than 6,000 words unless they have to, and, given the choice, most would sooner read two separate articles of 3,000 words each.

This means that you must know exactly how long your article is. An average quarto sheet in double-spaced typing holds about 250 words, and a foolscap sheet about 400. If you are in any doubt, get your secretary to do a more accurate check, not forgetting to allow for tables and illustrations, which often take up a lot of room. It is no good unloading a very long paper on an editor and expecting him to suggest where cuts should be made; this is comparable to the often-quoted 'please see and advise' referral note from a bad general practitioner to a consultant. If your bad manners are rewarded by the editor sending the article back by return of post, you have only yourself to blame.

The only care is that you must constantly check the length of your article. Go over the draft again and again, asking yourself what is superfluous and what is repetition. Put it away for three weeks and then read it again with a fresh, critical eye. Revise the draft and show the new typescript to a couple of critical colleagues (preferably in other specialties as well) for their advice on how it can be improved and shortened. Finally, ask a non-medical person for his views on the English style.

Shortness, simplicity, and clarity should be the aim of a scientific author. Too often, however, the article he writes reads something like this:

'A report is presented of the results of a controlled investigation of the therapeutic efficacy of minimising the manganese concentration in the dietary intake of ambulant cases with proven ulcerative proctocolitis. During a period of two years matched control and study case-material were assessed on a number of parameters. Among the study-group both utilisation and appreciation of the manganese-low diet was consistently high, a considerable proportion of them reporting that their spouses, siblings, and members of their peer-groups expressed readiness to consume manganese-low foodstuffs in order to minimise diversification in the meal preparation within each household unit. Both the study-group and the control cases were assessed on the basis of the differing incidence of absence from employment attributable to sickness. Among the low-manganese group, who totalled 31 during the course of the two-year investigation, the average number of days' absence attributable to sickness was 17.4 each year, while during the same period of assessment of two years patients in the control series (in whom the dietary regime employed specified low roughage, high calorie, high protein, low residue, and multivitamins) the average number of days' absence was 38.7 for each year. The nature and duration of exacerbations of the disease occurring in the two groups was also assessed. The authors concluded that among the group of patients on the minimal manganese regime (MMR) exacerbations were of reduced duration, the severity of the attacks was less marked, and the overall frequency was less, than among the controls.'

Many doctors would read this account without any comment on the style. Yet it is difficult to follow, and is four times as long as necessary. What could have been written is this:

'Exacerbations of ulcerative colitis are shorter, milder, and fewer among patients on a low-manganese diet. Patients like the diet, and for convenience their families often eat it too. A group of 31 patients treated with the diet for two years lost an average of 17.4 days off work per year, while among 34 patients in a matched group treated on an orthodox low-residue diet the average was 38.7 days per year.'

Why do editors not tell authors to rewrite their articles? Most of them are too polite to tell an author that he cannot write, and so they suggest only that the article should be shortened. The author of the summary printed above would probably shorten it as follows:

'A report is presented of a controlled investigation into the therapeutic effect of two dietary regimes in patients with ulcerative colitis. Two matched groups of patients were studied for two years, and the incidence, severity, and duration of the exacerbations of colitis experienced by the two groups were compared. Records were also kept of the frequency with which patients in the two groups were absent from work due to sickness.

The results of the investigation are discussed and recommendations made.'

This is worse than the original, which at least contained the important facts about the work. The author suffers from the two major faults of scientific writing—pomposity and jargon—and is unlikely to be cured unless he is prepared to spend time and effort learning the elements of a good style.

A doctor or scientist setting out to write his first paper and needing advice on style will find there is a wide range of books to help him. Some of the best known are included in Appendix E. There is, however, no easy way. You cannot learn overnight how to write well, and in practice few doctors are willing to write, revise, rewrite, and revise again solely to improve the presentation of an article. Most prefer to spend their time doing the clinical work or research, which they enjoy. Yet the subject is too important to be ignored or to take a defeatist attitude over; there are some simple guidelines for ensuring that you get your message across. If you follow them *and* get a senior colleague to criticise your draft, you will be on the right lines.

These guidelines aim at better scientific style and better English style. How you use them is your affair: I always find that I write gobbledegook but it is easy to rewrite a draft using the specific guidelines on scientific style and English style. The difficulty is getting the first draft, and transcribing something dictated into a tape-recorder may be the best answer. I am always struck by how clearly people talk and how pompously they write. If I asked you if you were doing any clinical research, you might reply: 'Yes, we've been trying indoxuridine in glandular fever. Interesting results—fever, cell count, and ESR normal within seven days, and they're fully fit in a fortnight.' Yet when you write the summary of your paper recording these results, you slip into long-winded, pompous obscurity:

'An investigation of the effects of exhibiting the anti-viral agent idoxuridine in patients suffering from glandular fever (EB virus infection, Paul Bunnel positive) is reported. The results demonstrated that normalisation of the pyrexia, the blood picture, and the sedimentation rate occurred in a high proportion of all patients within a seven-day period from the start of the therapy....'

So I would suggest that unless you find it easy to write a draft, you should try using a tape-recorder and then go over the typed draft using the guidelines given in the next two chapters.

7 Better Scientific Style

Why did you start, what did you do, what answer did you get, and what does it mean anyway? That is a logical order for a scientific paper.
Bradford Hill, A., *British Medical Journal*, 1965, **2**, 870

To try to dissociate the scientific style of an article from its English style is obviously artificial. I am doing it partly for convenience and partly because when revising any draft you will find it easier to go over each aspect in turn rather than dealing with both at the same time. In teaching scientific writing, authorities differ on whether the scientific aspects of style should be taught before the English ones. Some believe that really clear scientific thought must be translated into really clear English, and so the teacher should start with the former. From experience I do not believe this, but the argument is unimportant: as in the debate over the relative importance of the libretto or the music in opera, the answer is that the two aspects are inextricably linked. Even so, one thing is certain: bad work can never be made into a good article, however good the English style.

The structure of a scientific article only partly reflects the traditional scientific method (making an observation; checking its truth; making a hypothesis; testing the hypothesis); so some people have suggested that the article's traditional format should be replaced by something that reflects more closely what the author thought and did. The trouble about this idea is that this new type of article is even more difficult to write, and to read. I have seen several articles written in this style (nicknamed 'stream of consciousness' articles in the *B.M.J.* office), and found it exceptionally difficult to answer Bradford Hill's questions: why did you start; what did you do; what answer did you get; and what does it mean anyway? So there is a good case for keeping the traditional IMRAD (Introduction, Material and Methods, Results, and Discussion) format of a scientific article. This also helps the average reader, who is interested mainly in your summary and discussion and not in the details of your methods.

The summary

Although most articles now begin with a summary, I suspect that this section is usually written after the rest of the paper. By this time you are tired of the whole article and only want to be rid of it. This may explain why submitted summaries are almost universally bad, whatever the authority or capabilities of the author. All too often an editor will find out more about the work from a covering letter or from the first four sentences of the discussion than he will from a summary.

A typically bad summary might run—

'A trial of cadmium sulphate in subacute sclerosing myelitis is described. The difficulties in assessing the results are outlined, and brief descriptions of some of the side-effects of the drug are given. A plea is made for further, large-scale trials of this drug in this disease.'

This account ignores the four basic questions, and, since the title of your article is 'Cadmium Sulphate in Subacute Sclerosing Myelitis', your summary tells the reader absolutely nothing new. The result could be that he will not read the article or even cut it out for his collection. On the other hand, all this does not mean that the summary should be an 800-word mini-article. Summaries are seldom masterpieces, but they should be clear, crisp, and to the point. Unless the conclusions drawn are very individual, they are best written in indirect speech. The one above could be transformed to read—

'To confirm reports that cadmium salts might benefit patients with various neurological diseases, cadmium sulphate was given by mouth to twelve patients with subacute sclerosing myelitis. Nausea was found to be a dose-related side-effect, the maximum tolerated dose being 3 g a day. Seven patients improved appreciably and none got worse. Further controlled studies of this drug should be made.'

The introduction

Apart from the long-windedness that comes from inexperience in writing, excessive length is often due to an obsession with detail and repeating much of the introduction in the discussion section. In fact, for most journals the shorter the introduction, the better. What the reader wants to know is the answer to Bradford Hill's question: why did you start? If this cannot be said in a few sentences it is unlikely to have been worth doing. Except for the review journals, a long 'survey of the literature' is almost always out of place in this section; it belongs in the MD thesis, because the examiners expect it, or, heavily abbreviated, in the discussion section of the article. If you start with excessive length or detail in the introduction you will get between yourself and the reader, and who can blame him if he gives up before he gets to the article itself.

The sort of introduction that might coax him to read on is as follows—

'Exacerbations of ulcerative colitis are directly related to the amount of manganese in the diet (Bloom and Boylan, 1974). Manganese can be leached out of foodstuffs by centrifugation in an atmosphere of xenon, and we prepared manganese-free foods using this technique. We treated patients with longstanding ulcerative colitis with a low-manganese diet for two years, and compared our results with those in a matched control series on a conventional diet.'

Although no literary masterpiece, this passage of seventy-one words has already told the reader why and how you did the work. The least it should do is make him look at the end to see what your results were.

Material and methods

Most sections devoted to material and methods are far too long and detailed. They should aim mainly to answer the question: what did you do? Give the details only if the methods are original; otherwise quote the source. Even if you do describe the method, it is rarely necessary to detail the actual make of apparatus and chemicals used, the type of centrifuge used, or the pellets fed to the rats. The interested reader can write to you and find out these details for himself. Never mix comment with this section or with the Results.

The word 'material' should be used only in articles dealing with laboratory work or animal experiments. When your article deals with patients, the heading should be called 'Patients and Methods'. Never refer to your patients as 'case-material', as this suggests a physician of the old school who can scarcely wait for

36

the necropsy findings. You may often have to go into considerable detail of patients' histories, but rarely to the extent of giving whole strings of normal serum electrolytes and differential white-cell counts. Instead, use some phrases such as 'the relevant findings on investigation were as follows' or 'abnormal results were'. Most readers will automatically assume that you checked the WR and Kahn and the blood-urea concentration. If you have missed out any tests that are relevant, the editor will almost certainly raise this before your article is printed.

Case histories themselves are usually full of superfluous words: 'Examination revealed a pale, anxious young male subject', instead of 'He was a pale, anxious youth'. Remember also to go through this section in the same kind of order as you would in the Membership or Fellowship exams; in other words, history before findings, inspection before palpation. If you really have to give long and complex details of an unusual or new test, consider whether you should not put them in an appendix at the end of the article. If the work has entailed experiments on people, state early on that they were volunteers who gave their 'informed consent'.

Results

This section answers the question: what answer did you get? You should present the results in logical order, chronologically or in the order of the complexity of the test. Try to put as many results as possible into tables. Check that any numbers needed in the text agree with those in the table and figures. Most editors have a keen eye for this kind of discrepancy, and they will not be very impressed if you start saying that you studied serum-manganese concentration in four men and seven women when the tables and figures show these in four women and seven men.

Finally, check the statistics and do not quote statistical jargon unless it is correct and you can personally vouch for it.

Tables and figures

Many journals print some instructions to authors in each of their issues, and, though these rarely say anything about literary style, they are usually quite definite about the way in which they want tables and figures presented. So, if you intend to send an article to a particular journal you should follow any instructions it gives. If the journal does not print any instructions you may still be able to obtain some guidance by writing to the editor. The *Lancet* publishes a leaflet on 'Writing for the *Lancet*', while the *B.M.J.* publishes 'Instructions to authors' in the first issue of every year. In any case, you should always consult the Royal Society's *Advice on the Preparation of Scientific Papers*, which is particularly helpful about tables and figures.

Tables should be used to present facts in the clearest possible way. They should not repeat information that is already in the text. Resist the temptation to cram all the measurements you made into one or more tables. If the information in the table is confusing, then probably it should not be there at all. The following is an example of a bad table.

Pt	Wt	KJ	AJ	PR	Urea	Hb	WC	CSF
HJ	114	+ +	—	↑	76	90	12,000	5
LK	84	+	+ +	↕	114	78	10,500	117
PR	71	+ −	+	↑	84	105	8,000	81
UU	181	+ +	+ −	↕	71	61	7,000	36
RX	100	+	—	↓	78	87	9,000	19
JS	76	—	+ +	↓	100	104	10,000	1

This records values obtained from a series of tests done on six patients. The reader can make an informed guess at the meaning of each column, but even that does not help him much. It is more helpful to state that 'no consistent pattern of tendon reflexes was found' than to record a series of +, + +, + −, etc. without defining the symbols.

The information that you finally put into a table should be unambiguous. Spell out in full the variables measured—serum protein, mg/100 ml; serum alkaline phosphatase, King Armstrong Units. The editor may insert abbreviations if his housestyle uses them, but your manuscript must be clear. Do not include units in the body of the table.

If your paper has only one table you should not number it and should refer to it in the text as the Table; otherwise, each table should be numbered, usually in roman numerals. Every table should be typed on a separate sheet and should have a title; for example, 'Table III. Haemoglobin values at term and six weeks postnatal'. Patients should be described by letters or numbers, but not by their own initials. Anonymity must be preserved.

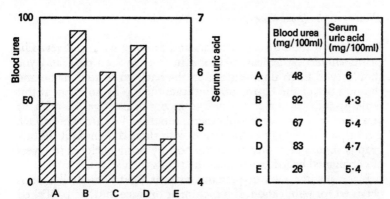

	Blood urea (mg/100ml)	Serum uric acid (mg/100ml)
A	48	6
B	92	4·3
C	67	5·4
D	83	4·7
E	26	5·4

Most graphs and histograms can be better expressed as tables. Which of the above is clearer?

Figures should also be used sparingly and for a definite purpose, which cannot be obtained with a table. A good example is the response of the various blood cells to treatment with different drugs in leukaemia. Most graphs and histograms can be better expressed as tables, as shown by the example. The advantage of tables is that the figures in them are accurate and that the reader does not have to use a ruler to find out the number of patients with a particular blood-sugar concentration. He can also check your results or recalculate them in another way.

If you have to use graphs, then get them drawn professionally. Look at the journal you are sending your paper to; measure the size of the graphs it prints; have yours drawn twice the size, on good quality board, in ink, with all lettering either written lightly in pencil on the figure itself or in ink on a transparent overlay. Before having the graphs drawn examine the journal's instructions to authors to find out the system of units it uses, or look at other papers it has printed on your subject. If in doubt use an accepted system, such as that published in the *Journal of Physiology*. Do not use symbols such as ϑ, Δ, Σ, or !! unless you have defined them in the text; they may be accepted conventions in a given specialty, but many symbols now have more than one meaning and confusion can arise. Always give the new data used in any graph in case an artist has to redraw it.

Photographs (half-tones)

Usually you should submit prints and not original negatives. The prints should be at least 6 in × 4 in (15 cm × 10 cm), and you should send them unmounted; on the back write your name and the number of the figure, and indicate the top by an arrow if this is necessary, using a soft pencil so as not to damage the print. If you want any part of the photograph outlined or arrowed, attach a transparent overlay to the figure with these drawn on it. Photographs should be protected in the post by being enclosed in layers of corrugated board larger than the prints themselves.

Black out the eyes of patients, even if their consent has been obtained for publication. If a picture of the face must be published without blacking out the eyes enclose a photocopy of the patient's written consent. Radiographs and photomicrographs can often be reproduced well only on special glossy art paper, but this depends on the quality of the paper used. The editor may be able to publish your illustrations on art paper, but usually he cannot. Select your illustrations with care, choosing those with the clearest features so that they will reproduce well on any type of paper.

Unless you use only one figure (in which case you should refer to it in your article as the Figure), your figures should be numbered, using arabic numerals. You should type captions for each figure on separate sheets of paper, which are then placed together with the tables at the end of the article after the references. Captions should be short (not more than fifty words) and should not repeat the text. Always give magnifications and staining methods in histological illustrations. If figures or tables are reproduced from other books or journals you must obtain copyright permission from the author and publisher.

Discussion

Most authors find the discussion as difficult to write as the summary. It is the one place where the IMRAD structure lets you down. Even so, there are some simple rules for the tyro. Write your discussion in short paragraphs. The first of these should sum up the replies to Bradford Hill's question: 'What answer did you get?' Later ones should answer his final question: 'and what does it mean anyway?' This is done by discussing your findings in the light of other reports. Finally, use your last paragraph to answer another question: 'and where am I going from here—to a larger survey, examination of one aspect of the problem, and so on?'

Look at the way the discussion is tackled in the journal you are sending the article to, and copy intelligently *if* you think it will help the reader. This treatment may subconsciously impress the editor, by suggesting that you have had some papers actually published already. But be careful: do not let the discussion get too long; it should never exceed half the length of the whole article and can usually be kept to a third of this.

References

The golden rule is to use only those references that are relevant and which you have read personally. Editors and referees are not impressed by strings of references, particularly when they are used to support statements that nobody would contest. 'Antibiotics have revolutionised the treatment of subacute bacterial endocarditis,[1-22]' is the kind of absurdity that alienates readers, unless the references are used to make a point. For example, if you mean that antibiotics are said to have revolutionised this treatment but in fact the improved prognosis is due entirely to better nursing, then a few references are acceptable. But remember the bathos that can be produced in Hamlet's speech which I once saw illustrated at a conference. 'To be[1-4] or not[5,6] to be,[7-10] that[8-9] is the question.[8-24]'

Sometimes you need to quote a reference you have read about in another article but are unable to read in the original. Here you should be honest and give both sources. 'Tyrrel, J, *Comptes Rendus de Zaire*, 1973, **2**, 456–8, cited by Fountain, R., in *Lancet*, 1975, ii, 10.' Work that has been accepted for publication should be described as 'in press'; that which is still being written up should be called 'in preparation'. Be sparing with the use of 'unpublished observations' and 'personal communication' for citing your own and others' work; both these formulae are overused and often give an article or letter the quality of Pseud's Corner.

References are one of those irritating aspects of articles where there are almost as many styles as are mathematically possible. There are two basic styles: firstly, the Harvard: Tyrell and Fountain (1971) in the text and Tyrell, J. and Fountain, A. (1971), Quantitative Aspects of Manganese Metabolism, *Quarterly Journal of Medicine*, 85, 2–5; and, secondly, superscript numbers in the text (with the numbers in the complete list of references arranged either in the order in which they appear in the text or in alphabetical order). With the Harvard system, all the names of the authors may be given every time or the first time the work is cited, or the words *et al.* used for the third (or fourth, or fifth) and subsequent authors.

This means that you must study the way the journal you choose cites its references. If you think that your article may go the round of journals, use the Harvard system; give all the authors' names initially and use *et al.* thereafter; and give a full bibliography in the list of references. In no part of scientific writing is agreement more urgent. I hope that the informal discussions now going on among a group of medical editors will soon settle this apparently trivial, but irritating and time-wasting question.

Abstract or summary?

For a long time different people have meant different things with the terms summary, synopsis, and abstract. Here I assume that synopsis consists of one or two sentences that do little more than indicate the article's content 'Manganese concentrations have been measured in various parts of the nervous system and their relevance to disease evaluated'. The summary is discussed on p. 35. Abstracts have usually been thought of as longer than the other two, giving more details of methods and results, and enabling them to be printed in abstracting journals without alteration.

A recent study by ELSE (European Life Sciences Editors) has suggested that editors should adopt uniform standards for abstracts, and that this term should be used in preference to summary or synopsis. Each journal should print brief guidelines for authors and provide back-up information on request.

The proposed brief guidelines are as follows:

'An abstract in English, of preferably not more than 200 words, should precede the text. It should convey the scope of the paper and give as much information as possible. It will normally *outline* the purpose and methods of the work, and *detail* important findings and conclusions. Further information on writing the abstract may be obtained from... The abstract is not an intrinsic part of the paper—it must be intelligible on its own, without reference to the main text. It should enable a reader to decide whether or not to read the paper; it should be suitable for filing and for use by abstracting journals. A good title and abstract help information services to publicise work rapidly and facilitate future retrieval. *Title and abstract are the keys to your work—write them accordingly.*'

No final decision has been taken on these recommendations, which are still being studied, but this is another section of the scientific article where authors and editors would welcome uniformity.

Title

An ideal title to a medical article demands the impossible: crispness that catches the eye and accuracy that tells what aspect of the problem you studied and how. Some journals partially solve this problem by having a main heading for the broad aspect of the article (often used for the 'running head' at the top of the pages as well) and a subsidiary heading for the details. Unfortunately, few of us can follow Richard Asher's example of good snappy titles: 'Myxoedematous madness', 'A woman with the stiff-man syndrome', and 'Why are medical journals so dull?' You have to remember that a reader in Stornoway or Alice Springs may decide whether to order a photostat from a library on your title which they read in *Current Contents* or *Index Medicus*, so that accuracy is preferable to brevity.

Many journals now ask for the name and address of the person to whom readers may write for information and for reprints, and it is a good idea to include these routinely in any article.

You should not forget to thank the people who have really helped you, including your advisers, technicians, colleagues whose patients you studied, and the patients or volunteers themselves if the study was an experimental one. One difficulty is, what qualifies people for inclusion in the list. A good rule is to thank anybody who has done more than the routine work for which they are employed. This includes the secretaries who type out your manuscript, which is hardly part of their N.H.S. duties. But avoid fulsome appreciations of your professor's help merely because you think that flattery will ensure you that next senior registrar appointment.

Who writes the article, and how?

Most articles carry the names of two or more authors; yet it is a recipe for disaster to sit around a committee table and write every word together. Either each author can write the draft of one or more sections, or one person can do the lot. The latter method usually produces a better article, which can be passed round for comments to the other 'authors'; one solution is to give this task to the person who did the least work on the project. But it is important that everybody approves, and signs, the final version.

Authors often ask about the 'best order' for writing an article. The answer depends on the writer and the type of article, but it is sound advice to begin by concentrating on the title, the summary, and the tables (how many; their design; their content). This method will expose any errors or omissions in the work itself, and provides a framework for the rest of the article.

Finally, remember that no article is likely to read well unless it has been through at least five revisions. Good writing is deceptively simple: as a former house physician of Richard Asher, I know how many drafts some of his best articles went through. Those who question whether the trouble is worth it should study the variorum editions of Yeats and Eliot, and imitate their continuing quest for the right word and phrase.

8 Better English Style

Good prose is like a window pane.

George Orwell, Collected Essays
Secker and Warburg, London, 1968

Any textbook of English grammar will tell you the six rules of writing clear correct English: choose the correct word; prefer the simple word to the pompous one; prefer the single word to the circumlocution; prefer the short word to the long; prefer the word derived from Anglo-Saxon to that derived from Romance; and use the active rather than the passive voice. Other sound advice is to use short simple sentences; write with nouns and verbs and not with adjectives and adverbs; and avoid the few obvious howlers such as floating participles and the less than happy constructions such as separating a subject too far from its verb. Using these rules you are well on the way to writing clear prose.

'I'm tired of grammarians,' some may say, 'language is a living thing; the meaning of words constantly shifts and anyway my message will be obvious to my readers.' But not all your readers are fluent in English, and, faced with an old word with a new meaning not yet given in the dictionary, a foreign reader may give up. Scientific writing should be as as accurate as scientific practice: the use of words with a score or more meanings (such as involve, marked, position, and situation) is laziness, a disinclination to worry over finding the word with the precise meaning you want. Finally, long pompous words destroy any sparkle or readability that your article might have had, and the non-committed browser stops reading. He may not know the reason for this, but if asked will say that it was heavy going.

Many of the best English writers have used short simple words and sentences, and no one would claim that George Orwell, for example, is any less an artist for having done so. In the preface to *The Playboy of the Western World*, J. M. Synge wrote that 'every speech should be as fully flavoured as a nut or apple', yet, in tragedy or comedy, his peasants, tinkers, and fishermen speak their moving lines in short sentences using short words. Of course, many great writers (including some great medical writers) have based their works on long words in complex sentences. Some, such as Shakespeare, have deliberately used the clash between Romance and Saxon to heighten their message. But these techniques are for the expert, and demand a lot of time. For most doctors who merely want to write a clear article with the minimum of trouble, sticking to the rules is the simplest course. If you would like to write really well, then you have a long but pleasant task ahead of you. Almost all great scientific writers such as William Boyd, Reginald Watson-Jones, or Peter Medawar have had a real interest in literature. Leisure time spent in reading for enjoyment will reward you by an appreciation of the qualities of good style, and in time this will be reflected in your own writing. Among well-known authors whose style has outstanding clarity are Conan Doyle, George Orwell, Graham Greene, and Peter Fleming. Not all fine writers make a good model for the scientific writer, however: an editor is unlikely to accept work modelled on the style of Samuel Beckett.

The six rules

In common with the other professions doctors like to mystify lay people, and one another. So they use long non-medical words which do not mean what they think. 'Anticipate', for example, means to take an action (as Gowers pointed out, the statement 'John and Mary anticipated marriage' means something different from 'John and Mary expected to get married'). The author usually means 'expect'. 'Mitigate' instead of 'militate' is another common howler, which schoolboys are expected to know for 'O' levels. So use enlarged rather than hypertrophied, unless you are certain that the cause of the enlargement is hypertrophy and not hyperplasia or infiltration, and use simple words such as chance rather than pretentious ones like serendipity. (There is a list of some commonly used long words and the shorter, better alternatives in Appendix B.)

This need to impress also explains why authors use pompous instead of simple words: why not, usually, say 'cause' instead of 'aetiology', 'treatment' instead of 'therapy', 'knee jerk' instead of 'patellar reflex'? Simple words are usually short and have a

Saxon origin, compared with the more pompous, longer words with a Romance origin—'start' instead of 'commence', 'gut' instead of 'gastrointestinal tract', and so on.

Much of the dead, artificial nature of medical writing is caused by turning sentences round, so that instead of saying 'We started treatment' an author writes 'Therapy was commenced' (or 'initiated' or any word other than started). Wolcott Gibbs described the effect of reading this sort of prose as 'backward ran sentences till reeled the mind'. Though it can be overdone, articles usually benefit from being written in the first person. Besides being more accurate, the use of 'I' or 'we' makes an article more readable, and nobody today will regard it as unnecessary self-advertisement. As the late Richard Asher, who wrote well and lucidly about the problems of medical writing, once said, 'Overconscientious anonymity can be overdone, as in the article by two authors which had a footnote, "Since this article was written, unfortunately one of us has died".'

Other troubles

A floating participle is one that has no noun to refer to in that sentence, the subject usually being understood. Some grammarians now accept that this construction may be allowed, but I still believe that it is slapdash and confuses the foreign reader. Interpreted literally, moreover, it may give ludicrous results: 'Having done a barium meal, the EMI-scans were reviewed again' implies that the EMI-scans did the barium meal. This is another argument for using the active voice, for this sentence would be better rewritten: 'Having done a barium meal, we reviewed the EMI scans again,' or, better: 'We did a barium meal and then reviewed the EMI scans again.'

The inexperienced often tend to pepper their sentences with subordinate clauses which separate the subject from its verb, or one main part of a sentence from another. This slows the reader and makes him work a lot harder. In the sentence, 'The elderly person with dementia, especially when they are transferred to unfamiliar surroundings, tends to wander aimlessly,' the main sentence is 'the elderly person with dementia tends to wander aimlessly.' The easier way of correcting this is to create two sentences out of one. Alternatively, the subordinate clause may be

brought to the beginning of the sentence 'Especially when they ...'
This exposes another common error in the original sentence—that
the pronoun in the subordinate clause is in the plural, the noun
and verb in the main sentence in the singular. Other similar
mistakes are to use a singular verb for two or more nouns, or a
plural verb when the true subject of the sentence is in the singular.
'The elderly man and woman with dementia, especially when
transferred to unfamiliar surroundings, tends to wander aimlessly.' But in, 'The elderly man or woman with dementia,
especially when transferred to unfamiliar surroundings, tend to
wander aimlessly' the word should be 'tends'.

Another error is to have the verb relating to the wrong noun.
The sentence, 'The accumulation of priorities, plans, and laws
mean that the hospital will not be built' is wrong: the noun
governing the verb is in the singular, and the sentence should be:
'The accumulation of priorities, plans, and laws means that the
hospital will not be built.' This is another reason for keeping
subject and verb close together, when this mistake is much less
likely to happen. 'Such a style is all right for Proust, though his
complexity has made me postpone reading him until I have
retired, but not for the tyro,' would be better written: 'Though
his complexity has made me postpone reading him until I have
retired, such a style is all right for Proust, but not for the tyro', or,
better, as two sentences: 'Such a style is all right for Proust, but
not for the tyro. Even so, his complexity has made me postpone
reading him until I have retired.'

Commas

The wrong use of commas is a frequent error and one of the more
important sources of confusion. Commas cannot be used in defining clauses but must be used in commenting clauses. So,
'Surgeons who cut themselves while operating often get streptococcal infections of the hands' refers to, or defines, only those
surgeons who cut themselves. 'Surgeons, who cut themselves
while operating, often get streptococcal infections of the hands' is
a comment and gives the sentence a totally different meaning: it
implies that all surgeons cut themselves while operating. In
writing sentences like this you should always ask whether you
mean to define or to comment.

Tightening sentences

One of the commonest causes of flabby writing is too many words. All of us have too many in our first draft, but we should then prune them vigorously. Common errors include the following—

Tautology: 'red *in colour*', 'round *in shape*', '*previously* described'.

Unneeded   'in the toddler-age child', instead of: 'in toddlers'. 'and
words: the fact that there is a slightly higher rate of pancreatitis is suggestive of the fact that', instead of: 'and the slightly higher rate of pancreatitis suggests that'.

Impersonal   I have suggested that you should always use the active voice
construction: when possible. Another way of improving your text is to alter sentences beginning with 'it'. So: 'It is only recently that definitive evidence has become available that', could be recast: 'Only recently has definitive evidence become available that'. 'It has been shown that in dogs hyperglycaemia may be produced by the injection of glucagon (Beetle, 1972). This fact is shown in Table IV', could be recast: 'In dogs hyperglycaemia may be produced by injecting glucagon (Beetle, 1972) (Table IV)', or 'Beetle (1972) showed that in dogs hyperglycaemia may be produced by injecting glucagon (Table IV)'.

Two verbs   The use of two verbs where one will do is a common cause
instead   of dead writing. 'A laparotomy was performed on the next
of one: day and the diagnosis of appendicitis was confirmed', may be rewritten: 'Laparotomy on the next day confirmed the diagnosis of appendicitis': 'Return of the serum cholesterol concentration occurs over a period of months', may be rewritten 'The serum cholestrol concentration returns to normal within months'.

In a spirited article in the *New England Journal of Medicine* Michael Crichton identified the recurring faults in medical articles: poor flow of ideas; verbiage; redundancy; repetition; wrong word; poor syntax; excessive abstraction; unnecessary complexity; excessive compression; and unnecessary qualification. Medical obfuscation, he argued, has become acceptable only in the twentieth century. It has led to outsiders having a low opinion of doctors; difficulties for doctors themselves in writing and reading medical articles; and a tendency of workers to read only papers in their own fields. 'But medicine is still too young, and its interrelations too poorly defined, to encourage premature fragmentation of knowledge. It is impossible to guess the cost here in wasted time, duplicated findings, and buried pearls.'

9 *How to Present Your Article*

Before submitting an article to a journal, an author should ask himself the following questions, at least: 'Have I something worthwhile to report? To what audience is this addressed? Have I made my point(s) clear and understandable for that audience? Is it entertaining (or at least readable) as well as instructive?' And last, but certainly not least: 'Am I saving my time at editorial expense, by not attending to the details of presentation?' If the answers to all these questions are favourable, the hopeful author may not be an Osler or a Churchill, but his paper will be published.

Ryan, P., cited by *Medical Journal of Australia*, 1973, **I**, 779

Care and time spent in the actual presentation of an article are well worth while. Obviously, if it is a rare piece of original thought with profound implications it does not matter if an article arrives as a poorly typed carbon copy covered with thumb-marks and tea stains, and without an accompanying letter. But regrettably such articles are few and far between. For the rest, the appearance and other features have a definite, if subconscious, effect in persuading an editor whether to accept it or not.

You must send the article to only one journal at a time. This restriction seems such an obvious courtesy, and also appears in every table of instruction to authors I have ever seen, that you might think it need not be emphasised. But every editor still gets about one article every year that eventually turns out to have been submitted to another journal at the same time. There may be rare exceptions to this rule—such as in the case of a Letter to the Editor asking for information or appealing on behalf of a charity —but you must ask the editor for his advice before you send anything for publication to another journal. This rule also applies to articles based on papers read to a society. Some of these, such as the Royal Society of Medicine, may want to publish the paper in their own proceedings, or in the book that gives a verbatim account of the conference, and they have prior claim. Hence you should always get the society's permission before you send your article elsewhere. But the fact that a paper has been presented to a conference does not prejudice its chances of being accepted if it fulfils the journal's criteria for acceptance. At the most, only a few hundred doctors are likely to have heard the paper, which in any case is likely to have to be rewritten for publication, possibly with additional material for which there was no time at the conference. In this case you should use the formula 'Based on a paper read to the Third International Conference on . . .'

The covering letter

Every article should be accompanied by a letter to the editor, even if you are a personal friend and have told him it would be coming, when you lunched together the week before. In fact, the more formally you submit your article, the better. If you write 'Dear Joe' to the editor, and three weeks later he has to turn your article down, he will be unable to look you in the eye the next time you meet, and your relationship will never be the same again. If they are to maintain the standards of their journals, editors have to be free to reject unsuitable articles from their best friends. But 'Dear Sir' puts the relationship on a proper professional footing, and will allow the editor to get one of his deputies to write you the rejection letter, if he feels that way. Similarly, if you are a junior doctor do not ask your chief to write a letter of recommendation to accompany your article. This will have no effect on the editor, who will judge your article entirely on its own merits.

It is always a good idea to say in your letter why you think this particular journal is the one in which your article should be printed. This advice applies particularly to general journals; good arguments here are to say that the work will interest people in many different disciplines, or that you want several other groups to try out this new method or drug to determine its precise role. Another approach that most editors cannot resist is to say that your work casts serious doubts on something already published in the journal, and that you want to put the record right; but make sure your thesis is watertight. Do not spoil your article's chances by saying that the journal has published several similar papers on this subject in the past year, and that you are sure the editor would like another, confirmatory one. Unless it is very good you will get it back by return of post, and rightly so.

Dual publication

Many journals ask for a statement in the covering letter that the material in the article is not 'already published' and that it is not being simultaneously submitted for publication elsewhere. The Council of Biology Editors considers any article that appears in the standard general or specialist journals (whether 'basic', 'applied', or 'clinical') is already published; material contained in published abstracts of papers presented or going to be presented at formal meetings is not.

The difficulty for the editor arises when a newspaper or magazine scoops a discovery announced at a scientific meeting, and the article submitted for formal publication adds nothing to this report: it is hard on the author if his article is rejected because a smart science correspondent has reported its message; but it is equally hard on a journal if the author has given a press conference on his findings, or supplied copies of his text and figures to the press, or both. The C.B.E. recommendation on this problem seems a wise compromise—

'Manuscripts submitted for publication that contain material that has appeared in any of the media described in the above two paragraphs may be considered 'already published' if: (a) the definitive article submitted adds no basic concept or important information to material appearing in one of the listed media (the addition of more data, greater detail, description of method, or more elaborate discussion does not necessarily remove the article from the category of 'already published'); (b) the definitive article submitted presents the same, or essentially the same, figures or tables as those published in the more limited communication or (c) identical paragraphs are used in both the limited and the definitive communications.'

If you want your article to be published with another one on the same subject by another author, try to arrange that the articles are submitted at the same time, or at least mention the existence of the other paper in your accompanying letter. Finally, the editor must be sure that the article does represent the views of all the named authors. For this reason many journals ask for a statement, signed by all of them, that they agree to publication.

Editors hate being bullied or harassed. So resist the temptation to telephone him or see him to find out whether he would be interested before you submit the article. Remember what it was like when you were a houseman trying to decide whether a patient had appendicitis or not from the GP's description on the telephone. Almost always you could only say, 'send him in'; the editor can only do the same. Similarly, unless the delay has been inordinately long, do not telephone to try to find out what is happening to your article. Almost certainly several people are reading it, and the reply to your query will be a formal one, such as 'we hope to write to you very soon', or 'your article is being read by an expert referee'.

It is good manners, though not essential, to write your article in the style of the journal you send it to. If the summaries in this journal come at the beginning of the articles, put yours there; if they normally print a 'running title' (that is, a shortened title at the top of the pages) or an address for reprint requests, give these; and try to list the references in the journal's house style. At present, journals have still not agreed about a universal 'correct' styling of references to previous publications. If you think that your article is likely to go to three or four journals before it is accepted, one way of avoiding having to change the style of references every time you resubmit it is to have several copies of a full bibliography made (*see* p. 42). Attach a new one to the back every time you have the article retyped. As well as the date, volume number, and the page number of the journal, this bibliography should give the full title of the paper, names and initials of all the authors, and the name of the journal in full. As with any quotations you may use in the text of your article, all these references should be carefully checked for scrupulous accuracy.

If you do not follow a journal's style, the editor will tend to think that you never read his journal, and are merely using it as a poor second or third choice.

Keep your manuscript tidy

Most secretaries in routine hospital departments are hopelessly overworked. This means they can type your article only in haste between the jobs they are paid to do. The final product is usually a bit skimped, and you will not be popular if you make a lot of corrections or ask for it to be entirely retyped. Until you are a professor or in private practice with your own secretary there is only one way to avoid these troubles: ask a secretary to do it outside office hours and pay her well for it. Find out what the going rate per hour is, and pay her double, plus something for materials. You will be surprised how much can be done in a couple of hours, and how impressive the finished product looks.

Avoid having any corrections at all in the top copy you send to the editor, which should be typed in double spacing on quarto paper with two-inch margins. Tables should be placed at the end of the article on separate sheets of paper. Figures and photographs, numbered and with your name on the back, should be put in a separate envelope, firmly attached to the typescript with a paper-clip. It is always a good idea to send at least one duplicate copy of the articles and figures, so that the editor has one himself for reference or can send the article to two separate referees at the same time.

When photographs and figures have already been published elsewhere you must get permission from both the author of the article and the editor of the journal (or the publisher of the book) in which it appeared. Enclose photostat copies of this permission when you submit the article, and mention the source of the illustration in your manuscript.

If your article is rejected do not expect to get it back in good condition. Although journals take great care of articles sent to them, almost invariably they have to staple the pages together and write a reference number on the title page and on the back of the figures. By the time a rejected article has been sent to and returned by an outside referee, and then sent back to you, it has been through the post at least four times, and usually looks it. For this reason many journals have now changed their policy of needing the top copy (and a duplicate) for making a decision: photostats are often now quite acceptable (certainly for the *British Medical Journal*) though it is a good idea to say in any covering letter that the original is available if the editor prefers it.

10 *What to Do if Your Article is Rejected*

Within medicine two sets of referees have recently been under fire. The first are the unfortunate individuals who are asked to review articles for publication in medical journals. The others are the people who are asked by authorities in charge of research departments to review applications for research grants. Since authors are seldom willing to admit that the product of their sweat and toil is anything but first-class, and since people with ideas for research are seldom willing to admit that their ideas might possibly have flaws in them, the stage is set for conflict.

Canadian Medical Association Journal, 1974, **III**, 897

More often than not, your paper will be returned by the editor of the first journal you send it to. It is natural to be depressed, but unnecessary. Remember after all that the same fate has befallen many articles that have subsequently become classical works.

Before you decide what to do next, remember why editors reject articles—usually on the advice of referees. They do this, mainly because the articles do not meet the criteria for publication or because they are unsuitable for their journal. A case report may be merely a 'me too', a long unoriginal account of a well-known condition that adds nothing to knowledge. The scientific method may be deficient, the statistical analysis wrong or bent, and the ethical aspects dubious. For a largely clinical journal the article may be too laboratory orientated, or vice versa, and in a subject that is split into many aspects (such as paediatrics) another journal may well be more suitable. In 'borderline articles' the editor and referee may be put off by the non-scientific aspects of the article: excessive length; repetition; poor flow of ideas; careless inconsistencies among tables, figures, and text; and gobbledegook. Given that space really is short, not surprisingly such articles are rejected in favour of the better written ones.

Logical approach

Once you have recovered from your disappointment that the article was rejected, go about things in a logical way. Read the editor's letter carefully: is it a polite brush-off or a sincere suggestion that you try another type of journal? If the latter, do you agree with the suggestion, and has the editor really understood why you originally chose his journal from all the others? Is a referee's report giving you a clue to the reasons for rejection enclosed?

If the letter is merely a polite rejection, you then have to decide what this really means. Either you think your article is some good or you do not. If you know in your heart of hearts that it is not good, you can hardly blame the editor for calling your bluff. By all means go on sending it down the social order of journals, for almost certainly you will get it published somewhere, but do not be surprised if first you get enough rejection slips to paper the bathroom.

If you still think your article deserves to be published, have another look at it. After all, probably by now at least a month has passed since you last saw it, and you may now see great deficiencies in your argument or your presentation. If not, next go through it carefully, considering the points discussed above. Is the article original, scientifically, statistically, and ethically sound, and sufficiently important for the particular journal? Is it too long? Are the Summary, Introduction, and Discussion absolutely clear? Is it well typed, or covered with corrections in handwriting and thumb-marks? Does it conform with the journal's format?

Ask your friends

You still do not know the reason why? Now is the time to ask a friend or two for their *frank*, and not particularly friendly, views. Pick one who is really familiar with the subject matter and another who has wide experience of successful publication and can advise you on the general impression made by your article. If both can honestly say that there is little wrong with it, tackle the editor himself. Perhaps he has a referee's report up his sleeve, which he has withheld for fear of hurting your feelings; ask to see this, and do not be offended if it more or less tells you that you know little about the subject. If the referee is right, then he was doing what he was asked to do. If he was wrong, you can point this out to the editor, but do this gently by letter, and not by trying to bully him personally in his office or on the telephone. These things should be done coldly and objectively, and any editor worth his salt will err on your side rather than the referee's. Most editors are willing to ask a second referee to have a look at your article for the second time, and it is usually up to you to say whether you would like this second opinion to be 'blind' or to take the first man's remarks and your riposte into account.

But perhaps the editor really was telling the truth and just has not the space for your article. He may have forgotten to suggest you send it to another type of journal, or he may be willing for you to turn it into a letter or a brief case report for his own journal. These things you may find out only if you write to him about the article. If you are perceptive you may also learn from the tone of his reply whether he thinks it has got any chance of being published at all, anywhere. But, remember, it is only his opinion, and it is well known that over the years many papers rejected by the *B.M.J.* have been accepted by the *Lancet*, and vice versa.

The moral is, therefore, go on trying, if you believe that the article is a good one. Never forget that the best work, wherever published, usually gets taken up by at least one of the general journals in an annotation or leading article. Also, do not forget that editors like to believe that they are the first to see an article, so remember to submit a fresh photostat or to get the manuscript retyped before you send it off again.

11 *What Happens to Your Article After it has been Accepted*

'I've read your novel,' he said. 'We'd like to publish it. Would it be possible for you to look in here at eleven?' My flu was gone in that moment and never returned.
Nothing in a novelist's life later can equal that moment—the acceptance of his first book. Triumph is unalloyed by any doubt of the future. Mounting the wide staircase in the elegant eighteenth-century house in Great Russell Street I could have no foreboding of the failures and frustrations of the next ten years.

Greene, Graham, *A Sort of Life*, Bodley Head, London, 1971

So now you have had a letter from the editor saying that he would like to publish your article. Where do you go from there? Two to one he has asked you to modify it in some way: to shorten it, to add something, to modify the argument in the discussion, or even to do some more work to make your case stronger. Do not fly off the handle at this. Almost always at least two people have read it, one of whom was certainly an authority on the subject. If they have misunderstood you, this is your fault because you have not been lucid enough. This means that you must consider any editorial objections or suggestions seriously. If you think they are wrong, ask some colleagues for their opinion. If all of you still think the editor and his colleagues are wrong, tell the editor so, but not by telephone because he is a busy man, will not readily remember your article in sufficient detail, and, anyway, will probably have to consult his expert adviser again before he can decide.

If the editor has asked you to shorten it, shorten it; do it yourself, and do not ask him to suggest the cuts. There are few things more irritating to an editor than prolonged haggling with an author, particularly when, as usually happens, his paper has been borderline anyway. It is embarrassing to be used as a continual postbox between the author and the adviser, and an editor would be less than human if he failed to admit that he cast a more than usually cold eye on any later paper this author sends in. (But do not misunderstand me; of course, any editor tries his best to help his author, to try to compromise, or to ask another adviser about the points at issue.)

Before the proofs come

Now that your article has been accepted, you can quote it, at meetings, or in anything else you may write, as Widmerpool, K., 'Cadmium sulphate in subacute sclerosing myelitis.' *Lancet*, 1977, in the press.

Once you have agreed with the editor on the final form of the manuscript, it should stay that way. The interpretation of your results, and any snags, should have been worked out before you sent the article to be considered at all. You will have a rough idea of the delay to be expected with the journal that has accepted your article. But even if this is several months, it does not mean that you are entitled to change your original text. If it is *vital* that you should change it, ring up the journal the minute you know, not the editor but his secretary, asking that the preparation of the proof should be held up. Follow this up immediately by a letter stating exactly what changes you want and why; this should enclose duplicate pages of the original text with the alterations made. Even so, these changes should normally be restricted to gross errors. They should *not* deal with other cases of the same disease you have seen since writing the article, or a key reference that has appeared in last week's *Nature*; possibly these can be incorporated as an Addendum, but this should be asked for only exceptionally.

Another well-known irritant is the man who presses for early publication. Of course, you want to see yourself in print; of course, you think that your article should take priority over others; of course, you are frightened that somebody else will publish a similar paper elsewhere. But what you forget is that the editor also shares these fears, and he is as interested in getting a scoop as you are. He may be delaying publication for a particular purpose, perhaps to link it with a similar article, or to have a leading article written round your piece. I particularly disapprove of the author who tells an editor that there is an American (or French, or Swedish) team doing the same work, and that he wants rapid publication to give the British priority. In practice this foreign article never seems to appear. Most British journals are recognised to be particularly rapid in their publication schedules, and I find this kind of chauvinistic appeal unattractive and unworthy of a great international profession. What is more, few articles are so world-shattering that readers even bother to look at the date of submission or of acceptance of an article, or anybody cares about five years later.

The whole subject of pressure for quick publication has been put into perspective by Charles Roland and Richard Kirkpatrick, who analysed various factors in the publication of 103 papers by workers from the Mayo Clinic. Three-quarters of the authors' time was spent in thinking about the project, doing the research, and writing the article. This preparation took an average of 29 months (range 3–233), compared with that for refereeing of just under 2 months. Over a third of papers had to be revised (just over 2½ months), and the delay from acceptance to publication was five months. Finally, the time lapse between hypothesis and publication varied according to the type of article: four years for basic science and clinical research articles; two years for case reports; and three years for literature reviews. Thus, research ideas are at least four years old (and a few are much older) when they appear in journals: 'even if editing and journal processing were instantaneous, the average research idea would be about 40 months old by the time it was read'.

Subediting

You can keep subediting time to a minimum by taking care when preparing your article. Subediting goes through several stages, and if a query arises at any of these the subeditor may have to contact the author, with a delay. These are the main questions any subeditor asks—

1. Has the author fulfilled all the editor's suggestions (such as shortening the article or making a point clearer)? If not, does the correspondence make it clear that this was agreed between them?
2. Do the figures add up to the same totals in the text, tables, and

illustrations; do the individual figures correspond in the various sections; if there are any apparent discrepancies, are these explained? Is there a reference to each table and illustration in the text?

3. Has copyright permission been obtained from the author and publisher to use illustrations, tables, or substantial verbatim quotations from articles (usually taken as over a tenth)? Does the back of any illustration indicate which is the top?

4. Has permission been obtained from the patient (or his parents) to use clinical photographs of the face where the eyes are not blacked out?

5. Do any histological illustrations give magnifications and staining methods?

6. Have the references been checked and are they in the journal's style? Are all the references mentioned in the text given in the reference list? Are there any references given in the list that are not mentioned in the text?

7. Are the abbreviations and units those used by the journal?

8. Have all the authors signed a letter to say that they agree to the article's being published?

Reading the proofs

The three basic rules of proof reading are rapidity, accuracy, and the minimum of alterations. Unless there are exceptional reasons, you should return the proofs within three days. This does not mean a cursory reading. You must go through every sentence on the proof and compare it with the original text. The easiest way of doing this is to have somebody reading the original text aloud while you read the proof. Some journals rewrite your text more than others, and when they do a lot of restyling it is particularly important that you are sure that your original meaning has not been altered. All journals have a 'house style', and if you find that your word 'questionnaire' or 'autopsy' have been replaced, respectively, by 'questionary' or 'necropsy', it is no use changing them back on the proof, because this will be unacceptable, and you will not usually even be told that the editor has altered it back again.

It is particularly important to scrutinise those parts of the article the sub-editor normally has to change, such as the figures (which will probably be relabelled, and sometimes redrawn) and the tables, which may be laid out differently.

All the authors of the article should read the proof thoroughly, and initial it, but only one person should make any necessary changes on the proof. This means that preliminary alterations may be made by any author in pencil, but that the final ones should be done in ink. The absolute minimum of changes should be made, since the reason for sending a proof is to confirm the literal accuracy of the text and not to alter its content. Even taking out a comma can cost 10p, and inserting a long word in place of a short one may mean that a whole paragraph will have to be reset in type—a very costly process, as you will find if you get charged for it, as you should be. If you have to change a word or a sentence, try to do it so that the overall number of letters is still the same; in other words, only one or two lines will have to be reset instead of ten or twenty. If the editor will allow them, extensive alterations should be done by a type-written sheet firmly stapled on to the proof sheet in question. If there is more than one of these they should be marked 'A', 'B', 'C', etc., and clear directions made on the proof where they should be printed by writing 'take in A'.

Changes on your proof should be made in ink, using the standard method—that is, by indicating in the text that a change should be made, but indicating in the margin of the proof the actual change. Some of the signs shown on p. 63 are taken from the booklet published by the British Standards Institution. If there are queries on the proof (for example, apparent inconsistencies between the tables and the text) answer them clearly, as otherwise this will delay publication. Remember, once your proof has been returned, that any further alterations are virtually impossible, extremely expensive, and highly damaging to the author's standing.

PROOF CORRECTION MARKS

Extracts from BS 5261 Part 2: 1976 are reproduced by permission of BSI, 2 Park Street, London W1A 2BS from whom complete copies can be obtained.

Instruction	Textual mark	Marginal mark
Correction ends	none	/ *
Leave unchanged	— — — —	
Insert new matter		new matter
Delete	he*d* or *head*	
Delete and close up	h*o*le or is*not* in	
Substitute words or character	*meet* or me*t*	new word or character
Substitute or insert character in superior position	gm² or gm	e.g.
Substitute or insert character in inferior position	CO₂ or CO	e.g.
Substitute or insert full point or decimal point	Indeed or end	⊙
Substitute or insert colon	.. ..	
Substitute or insert semi-colon	.. ..	;
Substitute or insert ellipsis	.. ..	•••
Start new paragraph		
Run on (no new paragraph)		

* This mark must follow every correction

12 Letters to the Editor

*A general journal ... nearly always includes a correspondence column.
Especially where the journal is a weekly, this section can become a dazzling
forum where jostle the faithful and the doubting, the primly orthodox and
the outrageously heterodox, the angry and the complacent, the brash and
the circumspect. Together they provide a giddy kaleidoscope at which the
reader may stare entranced or from which he may avert his gaze if the
light proves too sharp.*

Douglas Wilson, I., Address to the British Medical Association
Scientific Meeting, Hull, 1974

In an average week both the *British Medical Journal* and the
Lancet devote at least 12,000 words to letters to the editor, and
Nature has a large correspondence section for the biological
sciences. Each issue of these journals may contain a total of thirty-
five letters, contributed by some forty authors. For comparison,
a typical week's original articles (including case reports and preliminary reports) number about twelve, written by a total of fifty
authors. Since the other weekly and fortnightly medical journals
and magazines, both in Britain and abroad, also have correspondence columns, this means that the average doctor is as likely to
appear in print in this section as elsewhere in a general journal.
Moreover, the chances are much better, the rejection rate for
letters being much lower than for formal articles.

Editors like correspondence; it livens up the journal, shows that
people are reading it, and allows 'ordinary' doctors outside academic units to have their say. Most letters that are not libellous,
obscene, or merely repetitive get printed without delay. And they
are usually more fun to write: not for the letter writer the
straitjacket of the IMRAD structure—he is free to say what he
wants in his own way. But this does not mean that low standards
are acceptable. As with an original article, you must check your
facts and figures, and brevity coupled with some kind of logical
flow makes for easy reading.

Are your facts correct?

Letters that are in fact short articles or case reports should be presented with the same care as a full version, a point already discussed in Chapter 2. Yet for some reason doctors who would never think of writing anything that had not been fully checked in an article will do so in a letter. Too often they rely on memory for facts, quotations, or figures, and if these are seriously wrong the whole purpose of the letter may be destroyed. Usually, however, carelessly written letters are those commenting on an article or letter in an earlier issue. For example:

'*Sir*—Your leading article in last week's issue (20th February, p. 285) lays considerable stress on the recent steep rise in mortality from cancer of the lungs. You blame this largely on cigarette smoking, and yet ignore the role of diesel fumes, which, belching out from the poorly adjusted engines of lorries all over the country, expose every man, woman, or child to their harmful properties. Diesel fumes are known to be carcinogenic, and the incidence of lung cancer is closely related to traffic density. Only pressure from the oil companies stops the development and production of cheap, efficient, electric cars. Why don't you have the courage to bring these facts into the open? Even more important, Sir, you ignore a much more major epidemic of our times—namely, road accidents. Since last year in England and Wales many more people died in road accidents than from cancer of the lung; how can you possibly ignore the existence of this terrible, and potentially treatable, disaster situation?'

This is the kind of spirited stuff that editors like. Yet few would print it. The writer's statements are *ex cathedra*, unsupported by his own data or by references. Although an editor might allow you to make your point about diesel fumes—a point which, despite all the evidence to the contrary, may still fairly be debated—he could not let your final statement pass unchallenged. If you had only glanced at the Registrar-General's Statistics, you would have seen that in, say, 1967, 28,252 people died from lung cancer and 6,541 in road accidents. What is the editor to do? He could print the letter, hoping that its views will be shot down the next week, but this might not occur, and anyway the harm might have been done in the minds of those who know nothing about the subject. What is even worse, such a letter may be quoted in the lay newspapers as gospel truth; corrections are never news.

Should an editor waste his time writing to tell a letter writer that he has got his facts wrong? He will certainly not gain a friend by his honesty, nor is the author even likely to see his point of view. If some of the facts are right, should the editor salvage the letter by rewriting it? Again, his trouble will bring him no thanks and often only abuse. So most probably he will file it, saying nothing; in this way he may lose a subscriber, and will almost certainly be accused of suppressing discussion. All this means that, as a letter writer, you must check your facts rigorously and see that any quotations are completely accurate. If you are presenting a hypothesis, make this clear from the beginning of the letter.

Anger—and after

By all means write an angry letter, but do not post it, at least not until you have reread it the next day and preferably shown it to one or two friends who are outside the argument. Anger usually looks petty or contrived on the printed page. If you really want to be nasty it is better to use the rapier of sarcasm than the bludgeon of abuse, but be careful of libel. Is what you say: 'likely to lower the plaintiff in the estimation of right-thinking members of society generally, or damage him in a professional capacity?'* Many editors have an eagle eye for libel, and consult their legal advisers if they are in any doubt. But they may miss something, and, if they do, both you and the journal may be liable for heavy damages. Libel may occur in letters about scientific matters, but is much more likely in medicopolitical letters. An isolated general practitioner in the periphery may feel angry about his mileage allowance. He writes to the mythical giveaway journal *Family Doctor Weekly* about it:

'Sir Andrew Aguecheek has the effrontery to describe the new mileage allowance negotiated by the committee for Private Homeopathic Practitioners as a victory! My annual mileage is 10,000, and at the paltry sum of 5p a mile all I get is a pittance of £500. My car does 10 mpg, and tax, insurance, servicing, etc. bring the annual running costs up to £1,500. Surely Sir Andrew must agree that a Phantom III is the sort of car a reasonable practitioner could be expected to run. He should resign, making way for a younger man able to get to grips with the problem.'

* Lord Atkin in Sim *v*. Stretch (1936) 52. T.L.R. 669.

If such a letter arrives on press day just at the time to reinforce a leading article, it may be scrutinised less than adequately. The following week both the author and the publishers are surprised to receive a writ, pointing out that the clear implication of the letter is that Sir Andrew is too old to negotiate competently, thus gravely damaging his standing as a consultant physician. But a little forethought and care would have prevented the whole episode, which, however it ends, is bound to be expensive, if only in legal costs.

The need for structure

Just as a sonnet is more difficult to write than a canto, a letter to the editor may be trickier than an original article. To make their points in 300 or 500 words (the usual length), most letter writers need some sort of formal structure, even though this is much less obvious than in a formal original article. This will make the task of writing a lot easier and help the reader as well. State in your first sentence what you are talking about. Does it refer to a previous article or letter (in which case give the reference), or is it a statement about something in its own right? Next state your point of view: are you refuting a previous claim, or modifying it, and is your evidence personal experience or other people's published work? If you really need to give a case history, or use a figure, do so, but be brief and confine yourself to what is truly relevant. Resist the temptation to self-advertisement; leave out those ten references to papers all written by you as well as the more obvious statements that put you in a good light. Finally, sum up the position as you see it, and then stop. If the letter is being written by more than one author, see that all of them agree to the final text, and that all of them sign it.

There is usually little need to send a letter to the editor with a note requesting publication. Exceptions are when you want to give some private background information (this should be clearly marked 'not for publication'). You might, for example, want to explain that another journal has already refused this letter on certain grounds, or that you wish to take up a point from a journal that does not have a correspondence column. Another occasion is when you want to publish a letter anonymously. Most editors will allow this in the case of serving officers in the Armed Forces or civil servants, and very occasionally when the writer's job might be put in jeopardy. In such cases you must give your name and credentials in the background letter so that the editor can assess your difficulties.

Remember your manners

To be successful, letters must be published quickly, and editors realise this better than authors. It follows that there is usually a good reason for any delay in printing your letter. Space may really be short; your allegations may be repetitive, libellous, obscene, incorrect, or, if you have written it in longhand, illegible. Obscure references or quotations may have to be checked. Perhaps the editor is preparing a version of your letter that preserves the new points in it and discards others which have already been made in previous letters.

If your letter does not appear in a 'reasonable' time (which depends on the type of journal and the country of publication), there is no harm in asking why. But write a polite letter rather than telephone. You may be tempted to hector and threaten withdrawal of your subscription, but reminding an editor that indirectly you pay his salary is hardly good manners. Nor are you likely to be any more effective than a patient who tries the same argument to persuade his family doctor that he should prescribe some unessential item. Nobody has a right to get anything published, and letters to the editor are no exception. But, after all, editors are interested in good, outspoken, fighting letters, and your approach may be at fault if they decline to publish yours.

13 What Should the Family Doctor Write?

Do not forget there is a research laboratory greater even than the Cavendish, the streets, the homes, the factories in which common people pass their lives—there is the laboratory of him who adds to our knowledge of social medicine.

Major Greenwood, cited by Pemberton, J., in
Will Pickles of Wensleydale, Bles, London, 1970

General practitioners, looking back with envy to the days of Mackenzie and Pickles, may think they now have few opportunities to publish in the medical journals. But they are wrong. True, the days when the *Lancet, British Medical Journal,* or *Practitioner* would welcome a 3,000-word report on five patients with heart failure treated with digitalis are over, but there are now more opportunities for family doctors to write than ever before. General practitioners are still in an unrivalled position to study common conditions over a moderate period of time for comparatively little effort. Although a tenth of their patients may move every year they still have the unique advantage of a population that is relatively unselected. Really meaningful answers to the questions, 'who gets the common cold?' or 'who gets depression?' can be given only by a study based on general practice.

Today, research is becoming commoner and better organised through such agencies as the Royal College of General Practitioners. More and more experiments are going on in the organisation of general practice. Finally, compared with fifteen years ago, the family doctor now has many more journals to choose from, several specialising solely in his subject. Even so, the basic advice to any author applies just as strongly to general practitioners as to hospital doctors and academics: know what you want to say, say it briefly and clearly, and send it to the most suitable journal. Remember, as a general practitioner friend of mine said, that getting articles accepted by editors is a competitive affair. Family doctors get a very fair deal from editors, but they must see that their articles are up to standard. One way of doing this is to do what hospital doctors can do much more easily—seek advice from colleagues. Draw up a protocol before you begin any research. This should include the aims of the project, how these are to be achieved, how bias will be eliminated, the types of patients to be studied, the ethical aspects, and the proposed statistical analysis. Finally, you should draw up some sort of balance sheet to show that this work is likely to be worth the time, effort, and money, Send this protocol to several doctors with experience in the subject to get their views before you start on the work itself.

The detailed do's and don'ts for writing articles from general practice are little different from those in other disciplines in medicine. So what follows is an outline of the type of work a general practitioner might do as the basis for an article.

Research

In no part of medicine is meaningful research easy, but nowhere is it more difficult than in general practice. Even so, as a family doctor you have a unique opportunity to study what, for want of a better term, has been called the 'natural history' of disease. As one general practitioner with a distinguished record of research has said, 'we have the opportunity to determine whether hysterectomy condemns a woman to eventual death from hypertension; whether depressive illnesses always spare virgins; and whether vitiligo invariably indicates impaired glucose tolerance; and also to try to identify the many clinical associations we consistently overlook.'* Nevertheless, this kind of work demands scrupulous record-keeping for at least several years. Moreover, at the end of this time new developments may show up deficiencies in your data, or even overtake the work altogether.

Most doctors naturally want quick results and so there is a grave temptation to look for easy solutions, and the easiest 're-search' may seem to be a drug trial. If this is a carefully thought out study, with well-defined objectives and expert advice from the start, your results may be valuable. If, as is too frequently the case,

* Porter, A., *British Medical Journal*, 1969, 4, 296.

the trial is done on inadequate numbers, non-blind and non-controlled, your findings will be of value only to the firm that makes the drug. Any doctor can get the results of virtually any trial published somewhere, and these may then be quoted by the firm concerned as supporting extravagant advertising claims made in high-quality journals. The moral is clear. If you want to do drug trials on your own in general practice, get outside help, statistical as well as pharmacological, from an acknowledged expert. Reputable drug firms offer this sort of disinterested help, but beware of the less respectable ones.

An alternative is to take part in a group trial. This may offer the advantages of adequate numbers of subjects for statistical validity and expert planning to eliminate many inherent snags. But do ask a few questions before agreeing to take part. Are there sufficient doctors in the group, or possibly too many? Is the trial controlled in such a way that the results from different practices will be comparable? What about the ethical and statistical aspects? Who is sponsoring the trial, are the doctors paid for each patient entered, what is its main purpose—to advance knowledge or to provide facts for advertising? Has the group published any previous articles and how have these been received?

Practice organisation

Nowhere in the world are there so many experiments going on into the organisation of general practice as in Britain. Whatever the faults of the National Health Service, it has left family doctors with much freedom to arrange their practices as they like. Because of the relative shortage of family doctors and the rising standards of medical care, group practices and ancillary workers are now the rule, and general practice is humming with experiments concerning their proper part in the community health team. The infinite variations possible in the pattern of general practice provide innumerable subjects for articles, as for example, under the following headings—

1. Appointment systems.
2. Ancillary workers:
   nurses, midwives (or combined 'community nurses'), social workers, psychiatric social workers.

3. Diagnostic services:
   laboratory, ECG, radiology (all three on practice premises or at local hospital).
4. Group practice health centres:
   building and design, equipment, organisation.
5. Hospital:
   liaison with district hospital; use of consultants, in group practice or health centres; general practitioner beds, in district hospitals, community hospitals, general practitioner maternity units.
6. Management of particular illnesses:
   for example, home versus hospital care of myocardial infarction, and roadside care of patients injured in road traffic accidents.
7. Transport.
8. Audit, and various forms of record keeping (including Weed's Problem-orientated Medical Records)

Because of the current interest in such topics, articles dealing with any one of them are popular with editors. Even so, the same general rule applies here as to clinical work. If your contribution is really a 'first' on a particular subject, or if it reports results based on a very large experience, try a general journal first. If it is accepted you will get a large and international readership, so that doctors in other parts of the profession will get some idea of your problems. The *B.M.J.* and the *Lancet* have sections respectively called 'General Practice Observed' and 'Views of General Practice', and the former publishes occasional collections of these under the title of *The New General Practice*.

If your article repeats previous work or adds to it only in detail you have a choice: either of writing a letter to the editor of a general journal, or an article for a specialist journal such as the *Practitioner* or the *Journal of the Royal College of General Practitioners*. This will give you a large, knowledgeable readership of people interested in the same problem as yourself, and such articles often provoke correspondence between the author and other doctors doing similar work.

Case reports

Journals still want unusual case reports, but to avoid disappointment you must find a topic of interest and some originality, decide the form in which the article will be written, and select the most suitable journal. Yet again you must ask yourself: what am I aiming to do? Am I going to record something really new, to emphasise an unusual feature in the context of general practice, or to add to the small number of similar cases already reported? Here your main difficulty may be that what seems unique to you may be familiar small print to a hospital doctor. This does not necessarily mean that you should not write the article. If the features are sufficiently unusual or an effective reminder of the correct way of treating a life-threatening disease, an editor of a general journal might welcome a short letter or even a 600-word case report, while a specialist general practitioner journal might accept a fuller, more formal account.

In either event, your first step should be to look up the references on the subject, in the *Index Medicus* at your local postgraduate medical centre. Ask the postgraduate tutor or one of the local consultants for his reaction, or even write to an acknowledged expert on the subject. Above all, do make full notes at the time of seeing any patient whose features may be sufficiently interesting to be included in a future article.

Critical advice

Once your article is finished you should also do what every hospital doctor does—ask some colleagues for their critical comments. Either ask the doctors to whom you sent the protocol or try the article on somebody entirely new to your study. Try to get comments on the scientific and statistical aspects, as well as your English style and the layout.

14 *The MD Thesis*

Unlike an examination which is essentially a test of knowledge, pursuing an MD or a Ph.D by thesis judges a candidate's ability to investigate a problem in depth. The thesis must show a high standard of scientific and scholastic excellence and reveal, not only the candidate's knowledge of the subject, but his powers of deduction and reasoning. This involves a thorough study of the literature, careful recording and analysis of collected data, followed by discussion and conclusions, which show the candidate's complete command of the subject.

Williams, W. O., *British Journal of Medical Education*, 1969, **3**, 171

Any thesis is a formidable undertaking. Not only does it require time to do the original work, read other papers on the subject, and complete the actual writing, but the writer also needs stamina to keep at it over many months or even a few years, often together with treating patients or research. Moreover, at the end of it all there is often some sort of examination. Until recently an MD was required of applicants for most consultant posts in medicine, and I suspect that the strain of trying simultaneously to obtain this and having to do routine work was responsible for many people emigrating. But today many consultant physicians are appointed without having this degree, which is coming to be essential only for academic appointments, while those who want or have to write a thesis are much more readily granted study leave to do the research work and to write than before. Attachments to research departments in the U.S.A. are much more routine at the senior registrar stage than they used to be. Today, relatively fewer doctors are writing theses, and this is a pity because it is one of the best opportunities any doctor ever has of studying a subject in depth.

Because the pattern of thesis required for an MD varies according to the university concerned. I can deal only rather superficially with a few general principles. Also my remarks are necessarily second-hand: though I have rewritten a number of theses, I have never written one myself and this chapter is based on this experience as well as conversations with several examiners at various universities. It is a mistake, however, to start a thesis before you have some experience of writing and research. The preparation of one or two short articles or case reports inevitably forces an author to find his way round libraries and helps him to understand the principles of scientific method.

Preparation

The way in which you should approach the thesis is little different from that in an article. Having decided on your subject, and knowing that you have the means of doing it, you should start by asking: what am I trying to find out; what has been done before; and what is going on in this subject at present? You must contact your university as early as possible, to get a ruling on whether the work will be acceptable, whether a supervisor will be appointed, and what the nature of the examination will be. Normally you will be working in a department specialising in the subject and your chief will be able to answer these questions. But nobody is infallible and you would be foolish not to check very thoroughly yourself, using review articles, reference books, the *Index Medicus*, and your medical librarian as before. If you are going to write a thesis from outside a department and unsupervised (for example, from general practice), you should spend a good deal of time on these preliminary checks. Few things are more depressing than going it alone without any help or encouragement. Even worse, after a year's hard work, is realising that it can never lead to a thesis and you have wasted your time.

Formal structure

One of the differences between a journal article and a thesis is that finally the former has a logical shape. But the structure of a thesis depends on you, and you must constantly have a logical scheme in mind. The easiest way of creating a structure is to go to your university library, take out several successful theses, and copy down what they have done. Notice also the variations in length; the range of the number of figures and tables used; and whether

75

the university allows you to present 'accessories' such as strips, cassettes or gramophone records, colour transparencies, and reprints of your other articles—either related to the subject of the thesis or not.

As in journal articles, never mix comments with facts. This is why so many subheadings may be needed in the discussion section, so that you may consider each aspect of your findings in turn. A typical order might be as follows—

1. *Title page:* title, your name and degrees, and the year.
2. *Career:* some universities ask for a brief account of your career, with dates of degrees and diplomas.
3. *Outline of the work done:* object of the work and the method used (50 words).
4. *Summary:* a fairly full (400–500 words) account of your findings and conclusions.
5. *Survey of other publications:* in considerable depth, with everything relevant mentioned—even if later you show that some of the previous work was wrong.
6. *Material and methods:* include details of definitions and methods used; if either of these is at all unusual, it should be described in full.
7. *Patients studied:* case histories given here.
8. *Results:* given in chronological order or in order of complexity; this is the one place in medical writing where nobody minds if you repeat the results in table form and in figures.
9. *Discussions:* say briefly what you set out to do, and what you found, then discuss each topic under a separate heading; the main heading of each topic should be central in position, with subordinate headings as 'shoulder' (or side) in position.
10. *Conclusion:* a brief summing up, putting your present work into perspective.
11. *References:* titles should be given in full, and the Harvard system of citing references used—Stripling, J., and Jenkins, N. (1974). Cadmium Sulphate in Subacute Sclerosing Myelitis, *Quart J. Med.*, **64**, 952, or Aguecheek, A., and Belch, T. (1974). In Some Aspects of Cadmium Metabolism, ed. J. Malvolio. London.

Lastly, the final version must be read by several people, including the head of your department. One of these should be chosen because he is able to comment on the literary style and presentation of your thesis. You must not leave any obvious, answerable questions unanswered (otherwise an examiner may raise them), and the copies must be immaculately bound, in the style directed by your university.

Once your thesis has been accepted, you have a fairly rich source of journal articles and papers for conferences. But two words of warning. First, publish nothing before it has been accepted; I have known cases where a thesis was rejected because some of its findings had been published in a journal only a few weeks earlier. Secondly, do not be too greedy. An average thesis might yield one or two articles for a general journal, two or three for specialist ones, and a paper or two at a conference. If you try to get many more out of it, an editor may think you are spreading the jam a bit thinly. So when an editor sees an article on laboratory aspects of cadmium sulphate in subacute sclerosing myelitis, with a reference in the text saying that details of the patients and of the results of treatment will be dealt with in another, he tends either to suggest that the first article should go to a specialist journal or that the author should submit a revised article which contains all the aspects of his work.

15 Papers at Meetings

I recall A. M. Cooke [saying] ...: 'remember you are speaking to deaf morons' (modified for international conferences to 'deaf, foreign morons'). This advice was not in the least offensive, as it may sound. It emphasized that material which to you was familiar, even stale, was to your audience new and perhaps difficult.

Pyke, D. A., *British Medical Journal*, 1970, **1**, 420

Most medical meetings are dull. Many of the doctors who regularly attend them do so out of a sense of duty, to meet colleagues, or to start their holidays cheaply. The chief reason for this lies in that deadening phrase, 'reading a paper'. You should rarely *read* a paper, just as you should rarely read a speech. You should know by heart what you are going to say, yet be ready to introduce new sentences on the spur of the moment to deal with points made by other speakers. Through nervousness, or real lack of time for learning, you may sometimes have to read a script. This will not matter if the whole construction and content of your account are entirely different from an article written for publication. The following suggestions may sound trite and obvious, but they are rarely followed. If they were, there might be fewer empty seats or people asleep in the average conference hall.

The audience

Too few speakers consider the nature of their audiences. Occasionally at my local postgraduate medical centre (where the audience is a mixture of hospital staff and general practitioners) a visiting pundit gives a lecture that would do well for one of those marvellous, highbrow Ciba Symposia, but is as far above our heads as *Finnegans Wake* for the average novel reader. So you must ask yourself, is my audience specialist or general? Do they know anything about the subject or not, and if they do, how much? What am I supposed to be doing in this talk—providing intellectual stimulation, bringing the audience up to date, or getting registrars through the Membership? Does the whole audience understand English readily? Or should I speak slowly for them to get my meaning, or for simultaneous translation into other languages? Am I supposed to be introducing a discussion (in which case I must be short and provocative) or giving a formal contribution?

The paper

The entire pattern of your paper should depend on what you are asked to do. If you have to talk for an hour, then the paper can be in 'sonata' form: themes, exposition, development, recapitulation, and coda. The emphasis here should be on repetition, driving your points home in various ways.

But most contributors at conferences are limited to about ten minutes. One of these is lost at the beginning (people talking, coughing, and coming in late); another is taken up at the end summarising what you have said; and, if you show any slides, yet another may be lost in turning the lights up and down and in waiting for the next slide. So you have only about seven minutes to get your ideas across.

On the advice of educational psychologists, the B.B.C. recommends that only one new idea should be introduced every three minutes. In other words, you can put over a maximum of three ideas in a paper, which you may have flown over the Pole to give, or, perhaps even more exhaustingly, driven yourself in the rush-hour from the centre of London to a suburban postgraduate centre. But by careful planning you can make your journey worth while, and your paper a real contribution.

The first way of saving time is to plan the paper carefully. Some people think that they can talk 'off the cuff', particularly if the subject is one they specialise in, or if they are slightly contemptuous of their audience. This approach is not only arrogant; it is almost always a failure, resulting in long pauses, with 'ums' and 'errs' and the speaker forgetting important points which should have come at the beginning of the talk. Nobody would think of writing a paper or review article for publication in this way, so why should they try to do it for an audience? Most of the best speakers who appear to talk spontaneously at meetings spend hours in detailed planning, rewriting, and rehearsal. Whatever your audience, you should devote much time and effort to what you want to say.

Secondly, you should compare notes with the other speakers before the same meeting. All too often I hear this kind of opening sentence 'I was going to talk about the human blood-brain barrier for magnesium, but Dr Fafner has already dealt with the handling of magnesium in the bloodstream, and Dr Fasolt has told you about its role in cerebral metabolism. So they have really said everything that I was going to say in my paper.' Or, what is worse, the speaker may ignore everything that Fafner and Fasolt have already said and blunder on, sticking to his prepared script and repeating their contributions in another way. At one time, the chairman of any meeting was expected to arrange well before the meeting precisely what each contributor was going to cover, so that this confusion did not arise. Today few of them seem to think that they have any responsibility beyond uttering a few unctuous platitudes and introducing the speakers. So you must take the initiative in avoiding any overlap. Find out who will be speaking at the same session, and write asking them what they intend to say or, even better, send them your script and ask for copies of theirs.

Thirdly, you can save time by deliberately leaving some things out. This should be done with care, and only if there will be an opportunity for discussion at the end of the formal papers. Somebody in the audience or another speaker may raise the matter then, but if not there will often be an opportunity for you to mention it yourself.

Even so, if you do deliberately leave something out this should still be included in your formal script for publication in the conference proceedings (the only exception to this should be when the entire discussion is tape-recorded for publication). This may sound like cheating, but it is not. In fact it underlines the point that script for delivery to an audience should be entirely different from one intended for the printed page. The former should be human, even anecdotal (a good time for anecdotes is in the first minute, which otherwise tends to be wasted), in conversational style, and slanted to the audience in question. A printed paper, by contrast, should be formal, without any padding, and aimed only at the generality of readers of the conference proceedings or journal. To illustrate what I mean here is the same material presented in two different ways.

1. Paper for delivery at a conference

For a long time we've been interested in the relation between the level of *manganese** in the blood and the degree of *consciousness*. We came up against this question ten years ago when we admitted a patient to the ward with *hyper*-glycaemic coma who *didn't* come out of coma when we'd done all the usual treatments. Now one *obvious* diagnosis was that he'd had a small *bleed* into his brain—but we could find no signs confirming this suggestion. Of course, we also checked his *electrolytes*, and did the usual x-rays, but everything was negative. It was then that one of my research students showed me an article written by Nick Alberich, of Niebelheim. This paper described a diabetic whose *hyper*glycaemia *hadn't* got better until the *serum manganese level*, which they'd found to be *low*, was restored to normal by a drip of 2 *per cent* manganese chloride solution. Fortunately, at the time that we saw our patient, our university biochemistry lab. was getting interested in measuring serum manganese. We took them along a blood sample from *our* patient and they soon showed that he had a very low level—2.2 *Donner units*, compared with the normal range of *eight to ten*. This led us to study serum manganese pretty intensively. We looked at *twenty-one* patients with *hyper*glycaemic coma, at *twenty* with *hypo*glycaemic coma, at *fifty well-controlled* diabetics, and at *fifty non*-diabetics who were admitted with *cerebral haemorrhage*. We also studied *two hundred control* patients who were admitted to the surgical wards for *repair* of their *inguinal hernias*, but who were otherwise well. As far as possible, the control subjects were *matched* with our patients as regards age and sex. I would now like to talk about our results. The first slide shows. . . .

2. Article for printing in conference proceedings

In 1973 we found that many patients with hyperglycaemic coma resistant to treatment had low serum levels of manganese (Mime *et al.*, *1974*). Alberich *et al.* had recorded similar find-

* You should go through the paper for delivery marking the words to be stressed—the 'punch' lines, and those words that may be confused with similar ones (hypo- and hyper-, for example) and numbers.

ings in the same year. This paper reports the manganese levels found in 91 diabetics and changes resulting from treatment.

Patients and methods

Various categories of patients were studied, as follows: 21 patients with hyperglycaemic coma; 20 with hypoglycaemic coma; 50 diabetics who were well controlled by diet and soluble insulin; and 50 non-diabetics with cerebral haemorrhage. Two hundred patients, matched for age and sex, admitted for repair of inguinal hernia served as control subjects. Informed consent was obtained from patients or their relatives in every case.

Routine haematological and biochemical methods were done by the methods of Loge (1970) and Froh (1969), respectively. Serum manganese was determined by the method of Donner *et al.* (Donner, Loge, and Freia, 1968).

Slides

Most speakers rely too heavily on slides; frequently they may show fifteen or even twenty slides in their ten-minute session. (My personal record is of a research scientist who showed 54 electron-micrographs in 15 minutes.) Few seem to realise that the spoken word alone can make a major impact on an audience. Part of this attitude comes from propaganda for the latest cult of audiovisual aids. Obviously these do have some part to play in medical education of all kinds, but their role is much less important than enthusiasts are claiming. (Nobody denies that the blackboard has its uses, but equally nobody claims that it should replace the spoken or the written word.)

The speaker who opens with the words 'first slide, please' invariably gives his paper badly, however good its content may be. The rule should be to ask yourself, do I need slides at all? If I do, what is the purpose of each one? Slides should be used sparingly, and to make or reinforce particular points. To take an elementary example, it is obvious that a slide of a patient with Cushing's syndrome or of the electron-microscope appearances in chronic glomerulonephritis may be worth two hundred words of text or two minutes of speech. But a complicated graph full of data may take as much as a minute to understand properly, even when you as the speaker have explained what it means, as you should.

One of the few exceptions to the rule that slides should be used sparingly is when the language is English but the audience foreign. If you have slides prepared in their language, containing all your main facts, not only will they appreciate the courtesy, but they will also understand you a lot better.

The actual preparation of the slides should be left to an expert in a department of medical illustration.* Make up your mind exactly what you want included on each slide before you go and see him. Try to present the message as clearly and crisply as possible (few slides should contain over 25 words), and show your colleagues your drafts to see if they have any suggestions. Above all, check your slides carefully before they are shown at the conference to see if they are accurate and show what is wanted. If possible get all your slides projected in the empty lecture theatre so that you are sure that they are in the right order and not upside down. Practise looking at them from the angles you will be placed in at the conference hall. This means that slides must be planned and commissioned well in advance of the conference. If you give little notice you will be very unpopular with the medical artist, and if somebody more influential comes along just afterwards, also asking for a set of slides to be prepared, you may find that you have been put at the end of the queue; in fact, you may be lucky to get your slides before the conference begins.

Holding your audience

You will hold your audience's attention in four main ways. Firstly, start with an arresting, and if possible, provocative opening ('It is just not true that cigarette smoking is a cause of cancer of the lung') rather than a dreary recital of thanks to your hosts or your collaborators. A good way of thanking your colleagues is to put their names and appointments on a slide.

Secondly, aim at informality and a light conversational style. This is perfectly compatible with high intellectual standards. Vary

* Those who *have* to prepare their own slides will find much valuable advice in the leaflet prepared for the British Orthopaedic Association by the Department of Medical Illustration at the Westminster Hospital Medical School, London.

the pace of delivery, and the speaking tone, and look at your audience as if they were your friends and not cattle at a market. Thirdly, practise your paper intensively—with a tape-recorder, to your friends, and if possible in the hall itself. If with a written article your motto should be 'revise, revise, revise', with a paper for delivery it should be 'practise, practise, practise'. Remember that actual delivery takes 25 per cent longer than any rehearsal. Do find out about the hardware in the hall; a friend of mine once lectured in a mid-west American university town, only to be told at the end that few people in the audience had heard what he had said. He had mistaken a small black box for a microphone and spoken softly into it, whereas it was merely a machine for telling the projectionist about the slides; as he had no slides and the audience was too polite to tell him he was inaudible, he did not discover the mistake until too late.

Finally, try to be different from the other speakers, so that your contribution stands out. If you are given 20 minutes, take only 12; use a blackboard or an overhead projector rather than slides; if they make a good point, introduce features such as tape-recordings—or patients. If you have to use slides, try to concentrate them into one short section of your talk, preferably to summarise your ideas at the end, preceded by those life-enhancing words 'So, to sum up . . .'

Essential differences

Most talks fail because people fail to realise that, apart from their *aims*, speaking and writing are totally different. The types of *aim* and important differences in *structure*, *content*, and *delivery* are summarised in the four tables below.

Aims of Speaking and Writing
Original communication
Review:
undergraduate
postgraduate: general; specialist
Philosophical-pompous ('whither pancreatitis?')

Structure	Speaking	Writing
Introduction	30%	5–10%
Body	40%	40–60%
Discussion	20%	30–45%
Conclusions	10%	5%

Content	Speaking	Writing
Ideas	One every 3 minutes	Theoretically unlimited
Repetition	Considerable	Minimal
Padding	Considerable ('From the conclusions we are aware that')	None ('hence')
Style	Conversation, informal (I'm; isn't) Short sentences, punctuated by dashes Sentences are strengthened by beginning with 'but' or 'and' Few references or acknowledgements	Formal

Required number of references and acknowledgements |

Delivery	Speaking	Writing
Adaptability to audience	Maximal, according to circumstances	Limited
Arresting introduction	Desirable	Not always possible
Jokes	Desirable	Usually irrelevant
Visual aids	A few relevant slides	Minimum of tables and figures
Length	Finish early	Short as possible, but can reach limit allowed

16 Writing for the Experienced

For an author, the reading of his reviews, whether favorable or unfavorable, is one of the most disappointing experiences in life. He has been laboring for months or for years to focus some comprehensive vision or to make out some compelling case, and then finds his book discussed by persons who not only have not understood it, but do not even in some instances appear to have read it.
Wilson, Edmund, *Atlantic Monthly*, 1935, **155**, 674

Most of this book is intended to help the beginner write his first article or two. But I am often asked for advice by doctors who, though experienced writers of original articles, know little of what editors want when they ask them to referee papers, write leading articles or book reviews, or contribute to textbooks. Obviously, the editor's requirements vary enormously but the following are some general guidelines.

Refereeing articles

Most journals are firmly based on a policy of refereeing articles to outside assessors. Even expert editors cannot be expected to know all aspects of their subject and the help of referees is vital in maintaining standards of published work and educating authors. Some people have challenged the value of this system, holding that it delays publication and is open to abuse. I believe this attitude is wrong: time spent in refereeing is only a fraction of that from concept to publication (p. 60), and, provided the referees follow a code and the editor closely monitors their work, the drawbacks are negligible. To put it on a high plane, moreover, journals should be socially responsible: the press and television are always on the lookout for exciting stories, and, if these are based on claptrap that any expert would have spotted, the journal that employs no referees is performing a disservice to society.

Doctors, it is true, may well notice such errors for themselves, and may write to the journal to point these out. But corrections are never news, and the harm has been done. Lay people do not realise that most scientific articles are not a final statement of truth but merely a contribution to a debate. So if you are asked to be a referee remember this aspect of publication as well; for example, by suggesting in an otherwise good article that the author should be more careful in his conclusions if these are not justified by his evidence.

As an assessor the amount of help you get from the editor varies. Some merely ask you whether the article should be published; others enclose a long check list asking you to categorise various aspects of the article with a space for detailed comments. But all editors need to know at least four things. Is the article original (for the country or the world) or does it have qualities that outweigh this need; for example, an important review or a reminder of a neglected but curable condition? Is it scientifically sound (this covers not only the scientific methods, but the logic and statistical and ethical aspects)? Is it suitable for this journal, or more appropriate to another? Is it well written in clear crisp English and as brief as possible? Answering these questions is not as formidable as it sounds. Remember that you are being asked your opinion on the article as it stands, not on some ideal paper that only exists in your imagination.

To try to dispel any idea that referees may behave dishonestly, several bodies such as the Royal Society and the Council of Biological Editors have drawn up a code of guidelines for them. These emphasise that the unpublished manuscript is a privileged document; the referee should not discuss it with the author or anybody else without the editor's permission, or use it for his own research. He must assess it objectively, and declare if he has a personal antagonism to the work or its author, preferably returning the manuscript immediately so that the editors can have it assessed by somebody else. Refereeing should be quick (most assessors for the *British Medical Journal* return the paper within two weeks). Keep spite and abuse out of your report, at least that part of it intended for the author's eyes: there is nothing against enclosing with this report a confidential letter giving any background information that may be relevant. Do not write all over the manuscript; it still belongs to the author. If you are one of those who are never happy without subediting as you read, take a photostat copy, and send this with your comments when you return the original manuscript to the editor. If in your assessment you quote published work, give the full reference.

Finally, remember that your role is as an adviser and that it is the editor who decides whether to accept or reject an article for publication. He may have good reasons for not taking your advice, such as adverse or favourable comments from other referees, and if he is courteous he will tell you so. But most recommendations are followed, and it is impossible to overestimate the debt the scientific world owes to the hard work (usually unpaid and always anonymous) of scientific assessors.

Review and leading articles

If you think you are competent to write authoritatively on, say, electromyography, it is quite reasonable to write to an editor and offer to do so. He may already have an expert in this subject, but every editor likes to have more than one. If the editor asks you to write such an article, however, do not automatically agree to it. Ask yourself some questions first. Is the subject really in your field? If not, have you access to enough up-to-date journals to tackle the article? Avoid writing on subjects outside your own experience, for you may make embarrassing mistakes, and will not be given another chance. Can you meet the editor's deadline? If you have doubts, refuse by return of post, but ask for another chance later. Finally, do not do it unless you want to. Half-hearted work is immediately recognisable.

If you agree to write, bear in mind the readership of the journal. A review of the Zollinger-Ellison syndrome written for *Gut* will be very different to the one written for, say, the *Practitioner*. With rare exceptions, orthodox views are wanted, supported by published work if possible. Provocative, personal interpretations should be reserved for conferences or for unsolicited articles, unless both you and the editor have agreed beforehand to stir up controversy. Some journals do have special sections for speculation, variously called 'Points of View', 'Hypothesis', 'For Debate', and if you want to put over some controversial views you should submit a separate article to be considered under one of these headings. This does not mean that if a subject is controversial you should not say so, and even indicate which side the majority opinion is on, and why. One recognised way out of this is to use the conventional set of phrases, 'Some workers have claimed that...', 'Taking the opposite standpoint, other doctors have suggested that...', or 'At present most people in this field believe...'.

Everything that was said in the chapter on style applies even more strongly to review and leading articles. You will find that most editors will subedit your original draft to bring out your main points really clearly. Even so, you can help by care in preparing the draft. Solid slabs of type discourage the reader, so break up the text into short paragraphs, and the paragraphs into short sentences. A reader who is skimming through an article usually reads the first sentence of each paragraph, and continues further into the paragraph only if he is still interested. Cut out all the padding, and you will be surprised how much can be said in 600 words. A passage on the diagnosis of unexplained fever written by an inexperienced writer for general practitioners might read—

'Two important conditions it is essential to include in the differential diagnosis of unexplained pyrexia if the patient has recently been travelling outside this country are malaria and typhoid. The patient should be interrogated about his movements in the period immediately preceding the onset of his illness, and should clouding of consciousness have impaired his ability to give a clear account of himself or if he is unconscious the matter should not be dropped, his relatives must be sought out and interrogated along the same lines.' (87 words.)

This may be said thus—

'Malaria and typhoid must be considered in febrile patients who have been abroad recently. Either the patient or his relatives must be asked where he has been in recent weeks.' (30 words.)

Finally, plunge straight into your subject. If you are asked to write a 500-word account of the effect of CS gas on chronic bronchitis, do not start with a review of the published work on mustard gas and phosgene in the First World War. Any editor who knows his job will merely cross out your first two paragraphs setting the scene, and you will have wasted your time.

Book reviews

The first rule in reviewing a book is don't unless you have the time to assess it properly. Many reviewers skip through the chapter headings and list these and their authors with an occasional qualifying phrase: 'Dr Detterling describes the role of the EMI-scanner in the management of subdural haematoma.' Of course, any review must indicate the content of the book, but it should also assess its virtues and deficiencies: this can be done only by reading the book thoroughly and thinking whether it achieves its aim or not. So you should always say in your review for whom the book is suitable and whether it complements or replaces existing works.

Some book reviews may be major essays, as in the *Times Literary Supplement*, but usually all the editor wants is 150–400 words. Resist the impulse to nit-pick: it is unfair to any author to dismiss work that may have taken years because he has made a few minor errors. That does not mean that if a book is bad you should not say so; merely that it is important to keep a sense of proportion. Remember all the time that probably many more people are going to read your review than the book, so you have a responsibility to be fair to the author and the purchaser.

Textbooks and conference proceedings

Most textbooks are now written by several authors, and if you are asked to write a chapter or two ask for a careful brief. As at a conference, you need to know whom your message is aimed at (undergraduate or postgraduate, general or specialist audience) and to know exactly what the other contributors are going to deal with. Many editors now send a detailed framework not only of your own contribution, but also of the others, though you may have to ask them whether they have a maximum number of references they will let you use and whether you are allowed to use figures and tables. Keep to this brief for length and content, unless you agree on a different one. Above all, meet your deadline: there is nothing ruder in medical writing than being two years late with a chapter that quotes references up to the month you sent it in, while your poor punctual colleagues' contributions look dated (and are).

Almost all textbooks contain too many words—more even than journal articles. For various reasons, such as lack of time and the distinction of the authors, few textbook contributions get the pruning from their authors, colleagues, and subeditors they need. In particular, they are often vague when they talk of treatment, giving few details of choice of drugs and dose. What the reader needs to know is what drug(s) do you want? Why do you want it? When do you want it? How do you want it? How much do you want? When don't you want it? American books are much better than English in this respect.

Another job you may be asked to do is to edit the proceedings of a conference for publication. First, consider whether anybody will benefit from reading the printed transcript. Sometimes they will, as with a symposium of invited speakers, or of a small-scale conference with a definite aim. But often they will not, and it is a waste of time and money to slave at editing a mass of scripts given at a vast international jamboree that nobody will read. If you decide that publication is worth while, it must be rapid (6 to 8 months), and you must be able to co-operate closely with the publishers and the authors. Find out from the former how they are going to print the proceedings—by printing, IBM-typing, or photographing the contributors' original scripts (which will mean that these must have a uniform format); also how many illustrations and tables they can cope with. With your contributors it is a good rule to insist on having their manuscripts and illustrations prepared for publication, and not for the actual conference (p. 82), *before* the conference begins. Anybody who has tried to pursue an author who had retreated to South America immediately after the conference will agree with this. Otherwise, fix a stern deadline for receipt of the paper—say, a month—and if the author does not meet it do not delay publication, but add a note to say that he read this paper, but the script was not available. The mere threat of this is enough to make most authors produce their articles.

How much you subedit the articles will depend on the publishers, the authors' tolerance, and your own taste. But at the minimum you should aim to make all foreign articles intelligible to English readers and vice versa. Have a uniform house style throughout: if the publishers do not suggest one, follow the spelling in a standard work such as the *Oxford English Dictionary* or *Chambers Twentieth Century Dictionary*.

17 *Writing for Money*

Most doctors who enjoy writing and do it well can find an outlet for their work, but they usually get more pleasure than money from it—in Britain only about thirty doctors make a real living from medical writing. Nevertheless, if you get satisfaction from seeing your articles in print you can also earn enough to pay for a modest summer holiday each year.

Medical journals

Medical journals pay small fees to authors of commissioned articles of about £20 per 1,000 words in Britain, and slightly more if the article is unsigned. Usually, however, they rely on recognised authorities to write leaders, reviews, and revision articles. One way for a young doctor to break into this field is to write to the editor of the journal concerned, offering to report a conference he is to attend. Occasionally, particularly for meetings outside Britain, a journal would like a report, but it is not prepared to pay a reporter's expenses as well as fees; so the offer of a report from a participant is welcomed.

If the offer is accepted, discuss the length and content of the report with the editor, and read earlier conference reports in his journal. Most inexperienced reporters send in unsuitable copy—

'Professor Foppa (Padua, Italy) gave a stimulating account of his studies of the natural history of pneumoconiosis in marble miners. His serial radiographs were correlated with radioactive xenon studies. Professor Jenkins (Chicago, U.S.A.) described the effects of a new drug, butamol, in bronchitis. He had been very impressed with the relief of symptoms induced by the drug. He emphasised the importance of making objective measurements of lung function in studies of this kind, and gave details of the techniques used in his laboratory, which he claimed to be "the best equipped in the world".'

Such a report is suitable for a social diary, but is quite useless to those who were unable to attend the meeting and want more information. Facts are what they need—

'N. Jenkins (Chicago) had studied butamol in bronchitis. Respiratory function in 103 patients had been assessed by weekly estimates of peak flow, forced vital capacity, and $FEV_{0.75}$. When treated with butanol 1 g twice daily, the average peak flow improved from 240 to 380 cm^3/sec and the $FEV_{0.75}$ from 1.8 to 2.31. No significant change had been noted in pulse rate or blood pressure. Jenkins concluded that butamol had a truly selective effect on pulmonary beta receptors and would be of value in patients in whom tachycardia might be dangerous.'

Usually you will be writing conference reports for a journal or paper that is aimed at a large non-specialist audience; in Britain, for example, this might be the *Lancet, British Medical Journal, World Medicine,* or *Medical News.* So, unless the editor has instructed you otherwise, concentrate on the papers that present new findings, reviews of many cases, or advances in treatment of interest to the average doctor. Remember that three-quarters of the doctors reading papers at conferences have come because they thought they ought to or because their wives wanted to see Tokyo.

Accuracy

Few contributors to a large conference present really new work, and most of them get by with a rehash of a previously published paper, perhaps with some extra details added. All this means that you must be very selective. Avoid trying to mention everybody who spoke, and concentrate on the really interesting contributions. Often the discussion after a paper will contain the most stimulating material at a conference. If so, report it, but be scrupulous about the accuracy of what people said and their names. This sounds easy to achieve, but it may be difficult in a crowded, multilingual conference. In particular, an editor hates getting names wrong in a report, as their possessors invariably take offence out of all proportion to the seriousness of the mistake, and for the rest of their lives accuse that journal of inaccuracy in all its other sections. If in doubt, leave it out, or, if you must report an unknown contributor, use some phrase such as 'Another speaker from the floor . . .'

Finally, if you are given a deadline by the editor, keep to it. Really large or important conferences may be reported by several journals, and no editor likes seeing an account printed by a rival a week before he has received yours. Even if keeping the deadline means writing in a noisy hotel room in the early morning when you have a particularly bad hangover or an attack of traveller's diarrhoea, you should do it if you want to stay on the editor's books. Few journals will expect your report to be typewritten, but do print contributors' names in block capitals, and if possible send a conference programme along with the manuscript, so that names, dates, and other details can be checked.

Non-medical publications

Very few newspapers or magazines have a medically qualified correspondent. Usually, one staff writer covers science and medicine, and many large newspapers have a medical adviser they can turn to on special occasions. So there is some scope for a freelance medical journalist, but access to the big magazines or the national dailies is almost impossible for an unknown.

How do you go about writing for a newspaper if you want to? Probably your best chance lies with one of the provincial or local newspapers. Go and see the news editor if he shows any interest, and find out what he is after. If you send in some contributions, try to find out whether they are the sort of thing the paper wants, whether they are printed or not. Always discuss your ideas with the news editor first, since the paper may have covered the subject already or would like it tackled from a particular angle. Do not be surprised if many of your contributions are not printed, however enthusiastically they were received. News is a highly selective business of snap decisions about priorities, and most papers throw away all the 'overmatter' after they have gone to press.

If you are providing general news stories or commenting on current topics, you may find that your newspaper already gets a lot of medical news (taken mainly from the medical weeklies) syndicated by the London press agencies. One way of finding something 'new' for a story is to look at the other weekly journals published abroad, especially the *New England Journal*, the

Journal of the American Medical Association, and the Canadian and Australian journals (likely sources are the correspondence and news columns). Otherwise, the specialist journals may sometimes have an article of general interest, which nobody else has picked up. But remember that if you do take on this kind of writing you must retain a broad general interest in medicine, and that you must be prepared to take snap decisions, and write under pressure about 'hot' news items.

Popularisation of medicine for the lay public is not just a process of translating the main items in the *Lancet*, *Nature*, or the *British Medical Journal* into simple language. Important advances in medical science are not necessarily of interest to the public, and conversely, events which are run-of-the-mill for doctors may make good news stories. To be of lay interest any subject must be presented at a personal level. What does it mean to the individual reading the paper? A story about Parkinsonism, for example, might emphasise how common the disease is, and indicate the chances of a fit young adult developing it by the age of sixty.

Always include case histories if possible—

'Five years ago Jimmy Stripling (the name is not his real one) was manager of a large supermarket, ran a new Jaguar, and had a three-week holiday in Spain every summer. Then he got Parkinsonism. Within eighteen months he found it took him nearly an hour to dress and eat his breakfast. He could no longer drive his car; his speech became slurred and difficult to understand, and he lost his drive and enthusiasm. Unable to work for the past three years, he has had to sell first his car and then his house. Doctors told him that an operation might help, but he improved very little after "stereotactic surgery"—an operation deep inside the brain.'

Ethical problems

Quite often a doctor whose name gets into the lay newspapers because of a particular discovery is invited to write an article for them. But any doctor who writes for the lay public has obligations to his readers and to his colleagues which sometimes conflict. He should resist pressures to sensationalise advances in treatment. Seriously ill patients and their relatives clutch at straws, and it is irresponsible to suggest, say, that the latest cytotoxic drug offers 'new hope for leukaemia sufferers' or that a new operation will reverse the development of ischaemic heart disease. It must often be made clear that a novel technique or new drug is being studied only in recognised research units, and that local doctors can do nothing to help their patients get the new treatment.

Any medical writer should resist pressure to disclose the identity of patients or doctors, especially if he has got his information in the course of his professional work. Orthodox medical journals are well aware of the interest Fleet Street has in the identity of certain patients. For this reason the face is blacked out in any illustration and personal details are omitted even when a patient consents to publication.

Similarly, if an account for the popular press is based on published work, there may be a case for describing the authors as 'two Oxford physiologists' rather than giving their names. Research workers are often embarrassed by personal publicity, and their colleagues may not realise that they did not seek it.

Finally, there is the problem of signing articles. Any practising doctor who intends to make occasional contributions to the popular press should use a pseudonym. This minimises the risk of embarrassing conflicts with colleagues or patients, and also avoids the risk of being charged with 'unprofessional' advertising.

18 How Can Foreign Authors Help Themselves?

BILL WHIMSTER

It must be accepted as a fact that English is and will remain the principal scientific and medical vehicle of international communication. Certainly it will be so for communication with the largest body of relevant information in the world—that is, North America. The English-speaking doctors will therefore enjoy a unique advantage—that of not having to learn other languages. This type of privilege is likely to be considered tolerable only if the English-speaking communities show evidence of special interest in arriving at and carrying through mechanisms aimed at facilitating the flow of information from English into other languages.

Renold, A., *British Medical Journal*, 1973, **4,** 405

For several years I have been 'language supervisor' to *Annals of Clinical Research*, one of the journals produced in English by the Finnish Medical Society Duodecim. The society told me that my job was to make sure that the *Annals* articles did not sound foreign to readers whose native language was English. My qualifications for the task were not great: I had no special knowledge of English grammar and was not a professional subeditor or copy editor. But, since I had reported many meetings for the *British Medical Journal* and had also had papers accepted by medical journals, Duodecim thought that I had some sympathy for and understanding of the problems of foreign medical speakers and writers. They invited me to visit their beautiful country, and the least I could do in return was to try to be an efficient language supervisor.

I do not think that an author to whom English is not instinctive can, without tremendous effort, develop the instincts to make his writing sound infallibly English to English ears. Why should he? It should be quite easy to write the article and then to persuade some instinctive English speaker to make it sound English by changing a few inappropriate words and adjusting the word order.

Unfortunately, the foreign writer is not protected from all the mistakes native English authors make themselves. Indeed, the foreign writer is likely to make them grandly, with the feeling, having read much medical 'literature', that he is doing rather well. So the person who agrees to supervise the language is often faced with a much bigger task than making it just sound English. He may have to unravel many layers of obscurity to find what the author really means, and in the process he may change it, or even find that their is no logical message. It can be very embarrassing.

Also, unfortunately, there are no firm rules to guide foreign authors. Some books give lists of words and phrases to avoid but the foreigner may create bigger confusion by trying to avoid them. In any case, bans are an unnecessary limitation. No ban on an existing word can be absolute. Even if relative proscription is accepted and clearly explained, there will always be circumstances in which the banned expression is just right; for example, when you want to be pompous on purpose or to make a joke.

It is not helpful to study books on English grammar because ideas about English grammar are changing. *Grammar* by Frank Palmer (Pelican, 1971) is a clear guide to the traditional Latinist approach and its defects. It also outlines the ideas behind Bloomfield's *Structural Linguistics* and Chomsky's more recent *Transformational-Generative Grammar*.

In this uncertainty I have tried to create for myself a general method to apply to articles sent to me by the *Annals of Clinical Research*, articles which have been submitted to *Annals* from many countries and already considered suitable for publication by expert referees. More recently I have applied it to articles coming from other sources, particularly the Middle East.

Be your own subeditor

I now believe that much of what I do can be done by the author, either by himself or in collaboration with an interested colleague. If the colleague will ask the author to explain exactly in his own words what he means by each sentence, and even each word, the article will become steadily shorter and clearer as unnecessary words are crossed out and simple words and constructions replace complicated ones.

Articles that have had this time-consuming treatment, sometimes more than once, are much easier for an editor to accept and for a language supervisor to make sound English without changing the meaning. I would dearly like to do my supervising verbally with the author because to do it at a distance is always to risk offending him. Indeed, I try to make it clear that my changes are only suggestions, not Holy Writ, and I make them in pencil so that they can be rubbed out if the author disagrees with them. At the same time I do not hesitate to comment on the length, the layout, or the logic. I am also convinced that articles by English and American authors would *invariably* benefit from scrutiny by colleagues. Not only articles but many expensive medical books are far too long and turgid to read because they get no such treatment from their authors or publishers.

I appreciate that many articles submitted in English have been written in another language and then translated. The 'colleague treatment' can be applied to the draft in the original language and, if possible, to the English translation also. The translator should preferably be familiar with medical matters as well as with medical jargon in English; otherwise he is likely to change the meaning. Translators without medical knowledge certainly produce bizarre results. Usually, I think, the language supervisor can recognise such aberrations but they must cause some misunderstandings. Finally, I have no doubt that language supervisors for medical journals must be as instinctively at home with the whole of medicine as with English. It is difficult for anyone without a medical, or possibly paramedical, training to have the whole range of instincts required. Language supervision is a time-consuming business and therefore expensive.

Getting started

To get started the foreign author must produce a first draft. Most medical articles follow the IMRAD structure (p. 34), but the same principles apply to editorials and reviews. Some of these have been dealt with already in this book, but they are worth repeating. Each sentence should be short and simple. Subordinate clauses and phrases should be kept to a minimum. Paragraphs should include the sentences relating to one idea or concept. The author should avoid abbreviations. A recent paper had 'E.A.S.L.' without explanation. Even with explanation, 'erythrocyte sedimentation rate (E.S.R.)', for example, abbreviations are frustrating for readers, who have to keep looking back to find the meaning. This form of discourtesy to the reader is perpetuated because authors are too lazy to write the whole expression out every time. They feel justified because they think it saves the editor a little space. As a reader I quickly abandon such articles, so that the author's message fails to get to me.

Having prepared a suitable draft, not necessarily the first, the author is ready to do his language supervision, with or without his colleague. He should carefully examine each word in each sentence to decide if it is the right form of the right word to express his meaning. He must, of course, have already decided whether the article is intended for American or British English readers. For the American market he needs a general American dictionary such as *Webster*'s and an American medical dictionary such as *Dorland*, for British ones the *Concise Oxford Dictionary* and *McNalty*'s.

Many American English words today sound foreign to British readers although many others have been absorbed into what is now international medical jargon. For example, 'mastopathy' and 'pathosis' are in *Dorland* but not in *McNalty*. 'Mastopathia' does not appear in either dictionary and must be presumed not to exist. The foreign author must avoid words or forms of words which do not exist by checking in the appropriate dictionary. 'Fallacity', 'unprecise', 'evoluated', 'criterium', 'criterias', 'aggressivity', 'progradiate', 'isovolumic', 'neoplasmatic', 'pathognomonicity', coarsely-granulous', euthyreotic' , 'provosing', 'debuting', 'hourse' and 'subfebrility' are all non-existent words that I have seen recently.

Latin forms, such as 'prostatectomy ad modum Millin', 'morbus Menière', and 'ulcus ventriculi' are not used these days.

Some authors use unusual synonyms, such as 'semiology' for 'disease features'. They presumably obtain them from their own language/English dictionaries. But if the language supervisor can find the word and its meaning, he can easily substitute the more usual synonym.

Some words are commonly used incorrectly. Patients are not 'material', which is inanimate, nor 'patient material'. 'Possibility' is often used when 'opportunity' is meant: 'we would like a possibility to take further readings', for example. Technical words are frequently used out of context. For example in 'this drug has a wide spectrum of effects' ('effects' and 'affects' are also often used wrongly) 'spectrum' is used to mean 'range' but it is a technical word to do with light. 'Sophisticated' is often used in the sense of 'advanced' but it is derived from the Greek sect of Sophists, who were prepared to use any argument, however fallacious, to support their ideas. 'Significant' is a word with a technical statistical meaning and should not be used if that is not intended, as in 'there was no significant injury'.

Overtones

It is difficult for foreign authors to appreciate the overtones that some words have acquired. 'Caseation', for example, is not just a cheesy looking tissue, but has come to imply *tuberculous* necrosis. It should not be used unless the author is sure that he means 'tuberculous'. 'Denomination' and 'ordination' have an ecclesiastical flavour, so that 'cirrhosis and chronic hepatitis were included in the same denomination', and 'the ordination of wheelchairs' sound out of place. However, the language supervisor can change these, if he understands what is meant.

Some expressions are illogical: 'Roentgenological symptoms', 'findings occurred', 'stored until analysed by the assay kit', 'portal hepatitis indicates'. Others make the reader wonder if the author really means what he says: 'morphological differences caused by the method'. Yet others leave him in doubt: 'with rather constant morphology'.

As he is examining each word and checking its meaning, the author can also delete redundant words such as 'in colour', 'in size', 'in number' from such descriptions as 'red in colour' 'small in size', 'few in number', and pompous expressions such as 'adult human organism', which the reader has to waste time and concentration on translating for himself. Such superfluous verbiage may provide useful thinking space for listeners to the spoken word, but medical speaking and medical writing cannot be treated in the same way.

Whether the word is in the right form depends on the whole sentence. The simplest approach is to make sure that each sentence has a subject and a verb and to see if there is or should be or should not be an object for the verb.

The subject and the object of the sentence must be nouns or pronouns. The pronoun 'we' is now accepted by most journals as making the report more direct. Concrete nouns are best. Nouns formed from adjectives, such as 'diagnostics' and the noun form of the verb, the gerund, as in 'Eating is dangerous', may be permissible but can be confusing. 'Normalisation'—formed from 'to become normal'—is a noun form American editors would accept but British ones probably would not.

Many nouns need the definite article 'the' or the indefinite article 'a' or 'an' to sound English. The foreigner is more likely to be right if he puts them in than if he leaves them out. 'Systolic arterial pressure was measured' does not sound quite right; 'The systolic . . .' does.

A noun is often qualified or modified by one or more adjectives or adjectival clauses or phrases which 'tell you more about' the noun Sometimes there are so many adjectives that the noun is obscured. Other nouns are often used as adjectives. Then it may be difficult to decide which noun is the subject. The '-ing' form of the verb, already mentioned as the gerund or verb-noun, is also used as the participle or verb-adjective. As a participle the '-ing' form must qualify or modify a noun. In 'After assessing the results of the series, the patients were given the treatment', 'assessing' is being done, apparently, by 'the patients', which is surely not what was meant. All '-ing' words must therefore come under suspicion. If there is any doubt about their meaning they must be changed.

The author should examine each adjective critically to see if it is a necessary qualification. If it is necessary, is it clearer as a simple adjective, as an adjectival clause or phrase, or as another sentence? How is 'small (adjective) volume (noun) frequent (adjective) diluted (adjective) milk (noun) feeds (noun) were given' best expressed, for example?

Fortunately, in English, the articles and adjectives do not have to take account of the gender of their nouns. Apart from nouns which are obviously female or male, all other nouns are regarded as neuter. When a pronoun is needed 'it' or 'they' is the safest bet, but if in doubt, repeat the noun.

Problems with verbs

The verb, on the other hand, has to reflect whether the subject is singular or plural (not 'solitary' or 'plural', as one author wrote).

Subjects that end in 's' are not necessarily plural. For example, in 'This series of patients was analysed first', 'series' is the single subject. Note that 'patients', a plural noun, is not the subject, so the verb is not in its plural form.

Secondly, the verb has to reflect time. When the author is writing his report all the work that he has done is in the past—'In our series myocardial infarction was associated with hyponatraemia'. If he uses the present tense, in the discussion for example, 'Our finding that myocardial infarction is associated with hyponatraemia', the author will be taken to be saying that the association occurs more generally than in his series alone, so he must be sure that the evidence supports such a reading of his words.

The verb may be qualified by adverbs or adverbial phrases. These must be even more carefully scrutinised than adjectives because they are often less clearly qualifying the verb. Putting '-ly' on to an adjective is seldom a good idea—'this importantly influences the results', for example, does not work; and to start a sentence with 'interestingly' distracts attention from the more important words in the sentence and is needed no more than the pompous 'It is interesting that . . .' is needed. Many sentences fail to sound English because the adverbs are separated from the verb. Their place is *usually immediately* after the verb, or after the active part of the verb as in 'sauna baths are also taken in other countries'. Sometimes an adverb is deliberately put in a different position to alter the meaning. In the sentences:

The eye surgeons operated only at Guy's Hospital yesterday
The eye surgeons only operated at Guy's Hospital yesterday
The eye surgeons operated at Guy's Hospital only yesterday
Only the eye surgeons operated at Guy's Hospital yesterday

'only' is telling us something different about 'operated' in each sentence. The author who is not sure which to use should make his meaning clear in some other way. The language supervisor is unlikely to know which one he means.

To alter the emphasis is less easy in writing than in speaking but the first idea usually has the most impact:

The eye surgeons operated at Guy's Hospital yesterday.
At Guy's Hospital the eye surgeons operated yesterday.
Yesterday the eye surgeons operated at Guy's Hospital.

So the author must put his ideas in order of importance. He should not put the least important idea first. If he does, the reader may fail to realise which ideas the author regards as important.

Prepositions are the little words that join the subordinate parts of the sentence on to the main subject/verb part. They are often misused. Like things are compared *with* like; but unlike things are compared *to* each other. 'Since', a word to do with time, is often used when the author means 'because'. 'When' must also refer to time. 'Where' must refer to place.

Conjunctions are the words used to join more than one main subject/verb sentences together. Two sentences are often clearer than one conjoined pair, especially if the ideas are not closely related. For example: 'The eye surgeons operated at Guy's Hospital yesterday and an anaesthetic machine was found to be faulty.'

A second look

By now the author has examined all the words he has used, in their word classes—noun, pronoun, adjective, verb, adverb, preposition, and conjunction. Many superfluous words have been discarded. At this stage he can examine the remaining words again with two other thoughts in mind.

Are the verbs he has used in the active voice? The passive voice gives no life to the sentence. One after another they sap the reader's determination to extract the message. 'The rest of the group was characterised by . . .', 'the administration of proctolol was stopped . . .', the patients were subjected to radiotherapy . . .' for example. By making all his sentences active the author can also get ride of more obscurities. His meaning becomes clearer to himself.

Does each word, particularly each verb, have the correct emphasis, for example:

'The results indicated that . . .'
- — suggested —
- — proved —
- — implied —
- — showed —
- — revealed —

Each of these verbs has a different shade of meaning. Which one should he choose?

Eventually it seems that all the words are right. The final step is to see that the punctuation is right. The safest way is to use full stops and nothing else. Commas may be tricky.

'The patients, who took the tablets, all recovered'
'The patients who took the tablets all recovered'

Both these sentences are correct but have slightly different meanings. Either comma alone is meaningless—the language supervisor would not know whether to take it out or to put the other one in. Commas should be put between the items in a list but otherwise they cause so much confusion that the sentence should be reconstructed without them. Colons, semi-colons, dashes, and exclamation marks are for professional writers, concerned with style and mood. We are trying to convey information as quickly and effectively as possible from a busy mind in one country to busy minds in others. It is all wasted if the author is like 'The Mayo Clinic Authors', who, as one foreign author wrote, 'remained voluntarily in the vague, being confused . . .'.

A summary of steps for foreign authors to take—

1. Sort out the information to be transmitted into:
   (a) facts: patients, animals, specimens
              methods and techniques
              results
              other people's results
   (b) ideas: hypotheses to be tested
              conclusions from the facts
              speculations
2. Write a draft in sections according to the structure chosen, IMRAD or other, in short simple sentences, bearing in mind whether it is for American or British publication.
3. Remember that many of the articles which failed to convey their messages to you, failed not because you were ignorant or stupid but because they were not clearly written.
4. Check the existence and meaning of each word with the appropriate dictionary.
5. Check the position and form of each word in each sentence ('ing' words in particular).
6. Check that the sentences are grouped logically into paragraphs.

7. Apply the 'colleague treatment'. At the same time reconsider why you wrote the article in the first place, to see if you have succeeded in explaining your ideas to less committed readers.
8. Write the final draft and send it either to your chosen language supervisor or to the editor of your chosen journal.
9. Enjoy the elegant simplicity of your writing when you see it in print alongside the muddled efforts of your competitors.

Appendix A
Where to Send Your Article

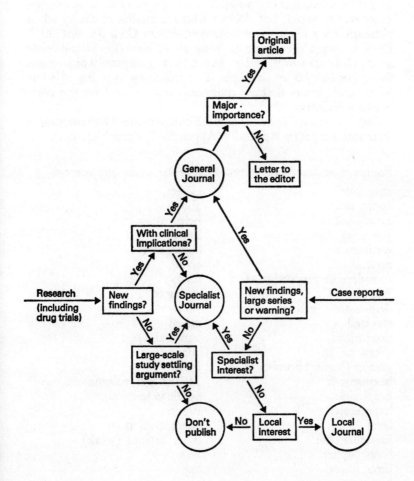

Appendix B   Words to Avoid

In a small book it is impossible to mention every word to use and every one to avoid. But doctors who are models of clarity when presenting a patient in person, relapse into Civil Servant 'high English' when they begin to write about him. Try to use fairly short, clear sentences and to avoid long, pompous words when there are simpler equivalents. The following is a list of some words and phrases that are commonly misused or have less pompous equivalents.

Some words are so awful and meaningless that I have separated them into a separate Appendix (Appendix C, Pseud's Corner).

Pompous or usually incorrect	*Simpler or usually correct*
anticipate	expect
approximately	about
assist (-ance)	help
author(s), the	I (we)
commence	begin, start
cervical collar	collar
considerable proportion of, a	many
due to	owing to
demonstrate, exhibit	show
elevated	raised
extremities	hands and feet
excess of, in	above
greater (higher) number of, a	more
haematocrit	packed cell volume
hospitalise	admit to hospital
hypothesise	suggest
level	concentration
literature, the	other articles (work)
limb, upper	arm
limb, lower	leg
large proportion of, a	much

Pompous or usually incorrect	*Simpler or usually correct*
large number of, a	many
majority of, the	most
mental patients	patients with mental disease
number of, a	several
outwith	outside
prior to	before
proportion of, a	some
regime	regimen
respectively	Use correctly: thus 'the blood urea in A, B, and C was 310, 515, and 125 mg/100 ml, respectively', *not* 'the blood urea in three patients was 310, 515, and 215 mg/100 ml, respectively'.
reveal	show
small number of, a	few
skin rash	rash
significantly	appreciably, definitely
sophisticated	advanced
sufficient number of	enough
through	up to and including
A and/or B	A or B, or both
in order to	to
it is apparent, therefore that	hence
it is possible (probable) that	possibly (probably)
it may, however, be noted	nevertheless
it may well be that	possibly
it seems to the present writer	I think
in the present communication	here

Appendix C Pseud's Corner

True, some of these words have a specific meaning (though not in the mainstream of medicine); but otherwise they are so awful that you use them at your peril.

attitudinal
cognitive
cohesive
colo/ileo-stomist
dichotomous
escalation
evaluative
global
heuristic
hierarchy
holistic
institutionalisation
interface
internalisation
intonational
kinesic
level (at the clinical level)
meaningful
methodology
modality
modular
multidimensional
multidisciplinary

normative
ongoing
overview
paradigm
parameter
particularistic
peer group
phenomenology
profile
quantitate
referents
remediation
seminal
situation
statementised
strategy
stratification
structured
symptomatology
to input
to output
universalistic

Appendix D Medical Ethics

In Britain, licences and legal controls apply to experiments on animals but not to clinical research. Recently, ethical problems have received more attention, especially in the light of unfavourable press publicity. Only in a very few cases, however, is there likely to be a real problem.

Therapeutic research

Research combined with treatment is ethical if it is justified by its therapeutic value for the patient. It cannot be ethical if it entails withholding the best treatment from the patient. It is justifiable to conduct a controlled trial of a new antibiotic in the treatment of meningitis only if, first, there is established evidence that the new drug is likely to be at least as effective as conventional treatment; and, secondly, that the control patients are treated with orthodox antibiotics.

Many investigators now use a prospective trial design which allows the trial to be stopped as soon as the results have reached a predetermined level of significance. Thus, if the new drug was better than the old for treating meningitis, this would show up earlier in the trial than if it was inferior to the conventional treatment; in the former case, the trial could be stopped at an earlier stage than the latter.

A trial that uses placebo treatment should be done only with the consent of the patients, and, indeed, consent should always be obtained if possible. Occasionally, it is not consistent with good management to ask for consent from a patient or his relatives as this might distress them. Patients with meningitis, for example, should not be asked to take part in a trial, and therefore the obligation on the investigator is more onerous. Non-therapeutic research, such as estimating the serum manganese in 200 patients with a hernia as part of a study of manganese metabolism, is ethical only if full and informed consent has been given by every patient.

Consent

It is not true, however, that any research is ethical if consent has been obtained. Four other conditions apply.

1. The doctor remains the protector of his patient's interests. If the patient has developed a close and dependent relation with his doctor he should not be asked to undergo any procedure that entails risk, as he is no longer fully competent to exercise choice; in rejecting the request he feels he has let the doctor down.
2. The patient must be fully capable of assessing the risk. Children and mental defectives cannot give consent (nor can others on their behalf) to any procedure that is unlikely to be of direct benefit to them. Ethical controlled trials using placebo therapy are almost impossible in children.
3. Any element of risk must clearly be explained to the patient, and the purpose and nature of all procedures described. The subjects must be free to withdraw from the experiment at any time.
4. Even if the risks are accepted by the subjects, the importance of the objective must be in proportion to the risks, and there should be an adequate background of scientifically established facts to justify the procedures. Non-therapeutic research should be done under the supervision of a clinician.

In 1964 the general ethical principles governing human experimentation were summarised by the World Medical Association in a code known as the Declaration of Helsinki. The full text of the code can be obtained from the W.M.A. or from the B.M.A.

Research Committees

Many institutions in the U.S.A. have research committees, and now in Britain on the recommendation of the Royal College of Physicians of London similar committees have been set up in most

British hospitals. If there is no committee to advise on the ethical aspects of projected research, a young doctor should seek advice from senior colleagues if he is in any doubt. Someone who can make an objective assessment should always be selected as the adviser.

Form of consent

If the research is of the kind that requires full and informed consent, it should be obtained in writing, and the fact should be recorded in the paper describing the work. Should some patients or subjects refuse consent, this fact should also be recorded. Finally, if the work is ethically objectionable then it should not be done. Many scientists may regret that, for example, cardiac catheterisation cannot be done on children unless this is essential for the management of their disease; but undoubtedly children cannot give consent to procedures which are of no direct relevance to their treatment, and their parents cannot and should not be asked to give consent on their behalf.

Appendix E Further Reading

1. Gowers, Sir Ernest (1964) *The Complete Plain Words.* H.M.S.O., London.
   A book on style for those who want to write simple, clear, and non-pompous English.
2. Fowler, H. W. (1965) *A Dictionary of Modern English Usage.* Revised by Sir Ernest Gowers. Clarendon, Oxford.
3. Bradford Hill, A. (1969) *Principles of Medical Statistics,* 8th Edition. The *Lancet,* London.
   The clearest exposition of the subject ever written.
4. Witts, L. J. (Editor) (1964) *Clinical Trials,* 2nd edition. Oxford University Press, London.
   A collection of essays dealing with the organisation of trials, and some of the snags involved.
5. Pappworth, M. H. (1967) *Human Guinea-Pigs: Experimentation on Man.* Routledge and Kegan Paul, London.
   Controversial discussion of ethical implications of clinical research.
6. Hawkins, C. F. (1967) *Speaking and Writing in Medicine.* Charles C. Thomas, Springfield, Ill.
   Covers speaking at meetings, symposia, and lectures as well as articles. Any doctor could read with profit the wise chapters on listening and talking to patients.
7. O'Connor, M., and Woodford, F. P. (1975) *Writing Scientific Papers in English,* Elsevier, North Holland.
   A clear, authoritative, and comprehensive account, written for scientists in general; highly recommended.
8. Calnan, J., and Barabas, A. (1973 and 1972) *Writing Medical Papers; Speaking at Medical Meetings.* Heinemann, London.
   Witty do-it-yourself books, written from the other side of the fence, for a change.

Nobody who writes anything should be without a dictionary such as the *Concise* or the *Shorter Oxford English Dictionary, Roget's Thesaurus,* and the *Oxford Dictionary of Quotations.* Finally, anybody who wants to see just how enjoyable a medical book written by a practising doctor can be should read *The Acute Abdomen for the Man on the Spot* (James Angel (1968) Pitman, London). This is one of the best examples I know where clear, simple language, together with a zest for the subject, can make a subject interesting even to those outside the field.

Index